STRESS ECHOCARDIOGRAPHY

Developments in Cardiovascular Medicine

VOLUME 149

The titles published in this series are listed at the end of this volume.

STRESS ECHOCARDIOGRAPHY
Its Role in the Diagnosis and Evaluation of Coronary Artery Disease

by

THOMAS H. MARWICK
Director of Cardiac Stress Imaging, Cleveland Clinic Foundation, Cleveland, Ohio, U.S.A.

Foreword by
William F. Armstrong

with contributions from
Jean-Marie Detry
Georges H. Mairesse
Jacques A. Melin
and
Jean-Louis Vanoverschelde

SPRINGER-SCIENCE+BUSINESS MEDIA, B.V.

Library of Congress Cataloging-in-Publication Data

Marwick, Thomas H.
Stress echocardiography : its role in the diagnosis and evaluation of coronary artery disease / by Thomas H. Marwick ; with contributions by Jean-Marie Detry ... [et al.].
p. cm. -- (Developments in cardiovascular medicine ; v. 149)
Includes index.
ISBN 978-94-010-4335-9 ISBN 978-94-011-0782-2 (eBook)
DOI 10.1007/978-94-011-0782-2
1. Stress echocardiography. 2. Coronary heart disease--Diagnosis. I. Detry, Jean-Marie R. II. Title. III. Series.
[DNLM: 1. Coronary Disease--ultrasonography. 2. Exercise Test. W1 DE997VME v. 149 1994 / WG 141.5.E2 M391s 1994]
RC683.5.S77M37 1994
616.1'207543--dc20
DNLM/DLC
for Library of Congress 93-41121

ISBN 978-94-010-4335-9

Printed on acid-free paper

This book is dedicated to my family.

Table of Contents

List of Contributors

William F. Armstrong, Director of the Echocardiography Laboratory, University of Michigan Medical Center, Ann Arbor, MI 48109-0022, U.S.A.

Jean-Marie Detry, Chief of Cardiology, St Luc University Hospital, University of Louvain Medical School, Brussels, B-1200 Belgium

Georges H. Mairesse, Research Fellow in Cardiology, St Luc University Hospital, University of Louvain Medical School, Brussels, B-1200 Belgium

Thomas H. Marwick, Director of Cardiac Stress Imaging, Cardiology Department F15, Cleveland Clinic Foundation, Cleveland, OH 44195, U.S.A.

Jacques A. Melin, Division of Nuclear Medicine, St Luc University Hospital, University of Louvain Medical School, Brussels, B-1200 Belgium

Jean-Louis Vanoverschelde, Division of Cardiology, St Luc University Hospital, University of Louvain Medical School, Brussels, B-1200 Belgium

Foreword

W. F. ARMSTRONG

While stress echocardiography is not the first technique to be applied to patients for the diagnosis of coronary artery disease, it represents an important clinical tool, likely to become of increasing pertinence in today's era of cost containment and mandated cost-effectiveness of diagnosis. It may be the most rapidly expanding area of clinical echocardiography today.

Stress echocardiography as we know it today represents the natural conclusion and merger of observations made over fifty years ago. In 1935 Tennant and Wiggers demonstrated that the immediate result of a coronary occlusion, was an instantaneous abnormality of wall motion [1]. As viewed from the surface of the heart in an open chest dog preparation, cyanosis and obvious paradoxical bulging of the left ventricular wall was noted. At a similar time Masters and co-workers, using fairly rudimentary exercise devices, described the response of the human cardiovascular system to sustained exercise (Figure 1) [2]. These two observations diverged for four decades while clinical investigation was pursued along the two parallel lines.

Following its birth with the Masters two-step test, formal cardiovascular stress testing evolved through a period of treadmill exercise testing or bicycle ergometry initially with one, then subsequently three, and finally twelve or more electrocardiographic lead monitoring. As the pool of patients being examined was expanded and the indications became more broad ranging, it became apparent that the symptomatic and electrocardiographic responses alone to physical exertion were insufficient for the diagnosis of coronary artery disease in many individuals and that accuracy could be refined and clinical utility expanded by adding cardiac imaging technique. The first imaging techniques to be utilized were based on radionuclide technology and involved either perfusion imaging with thallium or blood pool imaging with technetium labeled red blood cells. These techniques were developed and rapidly rose to pre-eminence in the late 1970's and early 1980's, they remain today the most widely utilized of the imaging techniques used in conjunction with cardiovascular stress. It was not until 1979 that echocardiographic imaging at the time of cardiovascular stress testing was proposed as a diagnostic technique (Figure 2) [3]. Following this initial encouraging, but obviously preliminary report, the technique essentially lay dormant. There are numerous reasons for this, including the technical limitations of early two-dimensional scanning devices, the lack of efficient mechanisms for data storage,

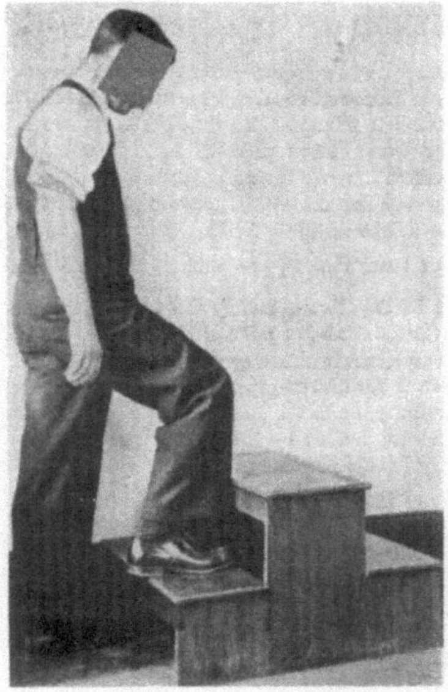

Figure 1. Illustration from the original article by Arthur Masters. Reprinted with permission of the American Heart Journal.

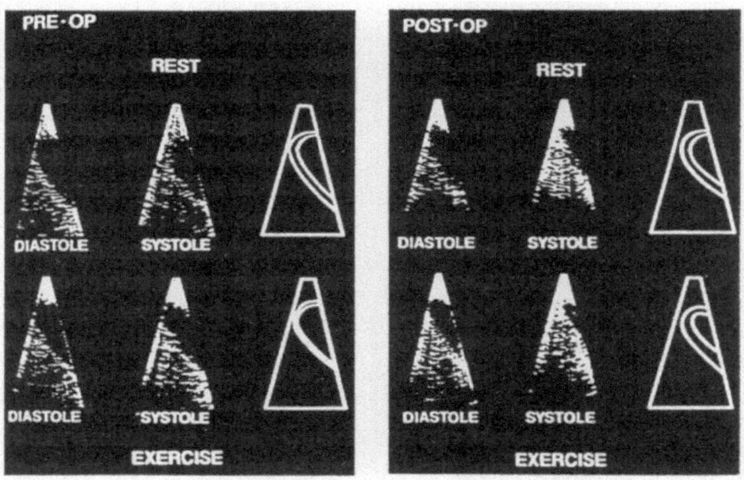

Figure 2. Early stress echocardiogram from the work of Wann *et al.* depicting a patient with significant coronary disease and inducible ischemia (left panels). Following successful bypass surgery there is return of normal function at rest and with stress in this individual (right panel). Reprinted with permission of the American Heart Association.

retrieval and analysis and the cumbersome nature of the examination itself. Finally the need for yet another imaging technique for diagnosing coronary disease was not firmly established, as the existing nuclear medicine techniques appeared then, and to a certain degree now, to be sufficient for clinical diagnosis. Fortunately the concept of stress echocardiography remained alive in the imagination of a small number of individuals who devoted substantial energy to further refinement of the technique, promoted its advantages and worked toward development of newer schemes for image storage and analysis.

In the mid to late 1980's multiple generations of ultrasound equipment evolved in a dramatically short time span, phenomenal progress was made in image quality, and with it an ability to image virtually all patients presenting for evaluation of coronary disease. Simultaneous with this we saw the emergence of digital echocardiographic techniques. These devices revolutionized echocardiography as we know it today, and allowed capture of continuous loop cycles for side-by-side display. It was this development, more than any other, which made stress echocardiography a truly practical examination. Combined with the improved imaging capability the digital acquisition devices made stress echocardiography a practical time-efficient and cost effective tool which could be applied to virtually all patients on an unselected basis as an efficient and accurate tool for the diagnosis of coronary artery disease.

What followed next was a virtual explosion of interest in stress echocardiography and in the number of laboratories actively pursuing it not only for investigational purposes but as a clinically relevant, practical patient management tool. As one laboratory after another reported results confirming the accuracy of the technique, often utilizing different forms of physical and pharmacologic stress, the enthusiasm for instituting programs in stress echocardiography dramatically increased. In the late 1980's and early 1990's "second generation" stress echocardiographers successfully disseminated the technique out of university based teaching institutions and into the community.

We now see an era in which a stress echocardiography laboratory has evolved into a common clinical presence, and with appropriate attention to training, a clinically relevant tool which provides levels of accuracy equivalent to that of the competing radionuclide techniques. It is not sufficient however to have a tool capable only of making a diagnosis; it is essential that the same technique be able to provide information regarding prognosis and patient management. Following establishment of accuracy for detection of coronary artery disease most laboratories have now turned their attention to the prognostic implications of stress echocardiographic responses. As we enter an era of cost containment, in which maximum clinical efficiency will be demanded, stress echocardiography, because of its tremendous versatility and accuracy for identifying patients with coronary disease as well as its ability to provide prognostic information is now poised as a leading technique

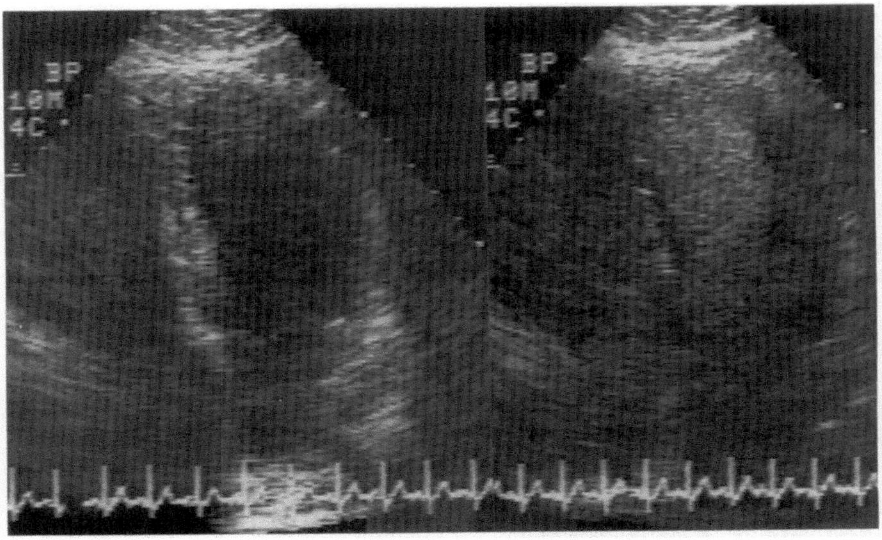

Figure 3. Apical four chamber view in an individual undergoing pharmacologic stress echocardiography. The blood pool has been opacified and the endocardial borders subsequently enhanced following an injection of intravenous sonicated Albumin solution.

in cardiology. The clinical utility has become well established and newer techniques show promise for potentially greater clinical and investigative uses (Figure 3).

In *Stress Echocardiography: Its Role in the Diagnosis and Evaluation of Coronary Artery Disease*, Dr. Marwick provides a thorough, comprehensive review of the basic and advanced concepts of stress echocardiography. This text represents an excellent starting point for individuals wishing to gain initial familiarity with stress echocardiography and a superb reference source for more experienced investigators and clinicians finding a need to further develop their understanding of the technique and advance its clinical relevance in their laboratories.

References

1. Tennant R, Wiggers CJ. The effect of coronary occlusion on myocardial contraction. Am J Physiology 1935;351–361.
2. Masters AM. The two-step test of myocardial function. Am Heart J 1935;495–510.
3. Wann LS, Faris JV, Childress RH, Dillon JC, Weyman AE, Feigenbaum H. Exercise cross-sectional echocardiography in ischemic heart disease. Circulation 1979;60:1300–1308.

Preface

Stress echocardiography is a conceptually simple technique which permits the detection of ischemic myocardium by direct visualization of the regional left ventricular dysfunction, which occurs as a consequence of ischemia. However, the simplicity of this concept contrasts with the technical difficulty posed by the practical performance of this technique, a fact well evidenced by the delay between the initial reports of this method by researchers in the late 1970's, and the relatively recent clinical interest in the approach.

The aim of this work is to investigate the application of this method as a routine diagnostic tool for detection of the presence, site and extent of myocardial ischemia. To this end, the pathophysiologic aspects which determine the development of abnormal regional function due to ischemia, and the ability of ultrasound to detect abnormal function, are reviewed in chapter 1. The methodology of the test and its interpretation are discussed in chapter 2. The subsequent sections deal with the feasibility and accuracy of exercise stress echocardiography (chapter 3) and pharmacologic stress echocardiography (chapters 4 and 5). Chapters 6 and 7 place stress echocardiography in perspective with reference to the currently available alternatives for the diagnosis of coronary artery disease (the stress electrocardiogram and nuclear scintigraphy). The use of the technique for purposes unrelated to the diagnosis of coronary disease – assessment of prognosis (chapter 8), evaluation of the efficacy of therapeutic endevours (chapter 9) and the detection of viable myocardium (chapter 10) are discussed in the last section.

Stress echocardiography is a technically demanding technique, both to perform and to interpret. While there is no substitute for "hands-on" (preferably supervised) training, the purpose of this book is to facilitate the acquisition of this expertise.

Thomas Marwick,
Cleveland, October 1993.

T.H. Marwick, Stress Echocardiography, xv, 1994.

Acknowledgements

This book represents a synthesis of work initiated at the Cleveland Clinic Foundation, Cleveland, Ohio, and continued at the St. Luc University Hospital, Brussels, during my period as Visiting Professor during 1991 and 1992. Its fruition reflects in large part, the support of Professor JM Detry, Dr JA Melin, and Dr W Wyns, who first invited me to work at the Catholic University of Louvain. This work has also been benefitted by the interest and constructive criticism of Professor J Roelandt and Dr P Fioretti, of the Thoraxcenter, Rotterdam, and the patient guidance of H Liepman and N Dekker, at Kluwer Academic Publishers.

I wish to particularly thank Drs S Woodhouse, P Harris, E Salcedo and W Stewart, who guided my training as a cardiologist and echocardiographer, and gave me the freedom to develop my interests in stress echocardiography. I would like to add a special note of thanks to B Haluska, J Nemec, J Torelli, T Baudhuin, G Mairesse, K Lee and J Williams – colleagues whose intellectual curiosity gave the impetus to many of the studies in this text. Finally, my wife and children deserve a great accolade for their patience during the long gestation of this work.

1. Basic Considerations in the Pathophysiology and Detection of Ischemic Left Ventricular Dysfunction

G.H. MAIRESSE and T. MARWICK

Regional systolic dysfunction is a very early sequel to the development of myocardial ischemia. Because of the ability of echocardiography to visualize the function of the heart non-invasively and in real-time, its use for the detection of myocardial ischemia has been the source of research activity since the earliest days of the technique. This chapter reviews aspects of function in the normal and ischemic heart, as well as imaging considerations, which are central to the understanding of stress echocardiography.

1.1 Pathophysiology of Ischemic Left Ventricular Dysfunction

1.1.1 *Normal Contractile Properties of the Myocyte*

Normal contractile function in the heart is intimately related to the behavior of intracellular calcium (Ca^{2+}). During cellular depolarization, Ca^{2+} flows into the cytoplasm, inhibiting the binding of actin with troponin and therefore permitting actin-myosin binding [1]. The resultant cross-bridge formation induces a change in orientation of the myosin head, thereby producing a relative change in position between filaments and cells, causing myocardial contraction – visualized at echocardiography as myocardial thickening and endocardial excursion. Finally, at the end of systole, the concentration of Ca^{2+} falls, allowing troponin to again bind with actin, resulting in relaxation [2]. Both the augmentation and the reduction of Ca^{2+} require energy, so that ischemia may not only compromise contraction but also cause abnormal relaxation (both of which are potentially detectable by echocardiography). In summary, the mechanical functions of the heart correlate with the quantity of Ca^{2+} which is bound to troponin and the myofibrillar sensitivity to Ca^{2+} [3].

The energy required for cross-bridge formation is derived from the hydrolysis of a molecule of adenosine triphosphate (ATP). Thus, when cardiac workload increases, due to increases of heart rate, contractility or load, the hydrolysis of ATP must increase simultaneously. Under normal circumstances, most of the heart's ATP is produced by aerobic metabolism [4]. Although oxidative phosphorylation is the dominant source of ATP [5], a variety of substrates can be metabolized by the cardiac myocytes, depending

T.H. Marwick, Stress Echocardiography, 1–10.

on their availability and the metabolic status of the heart. The major role of aerobic metabolism in myocardial energy production causes myocardial oxygen consumption (MVO_2) to represent the global metabolic activity of the heart, and as only 10 to 20% of this oxygen is used for physiologic processes not directly associated with contraction, oxygen consumption effectively correlates with cardiac work. The three main determinants of MVO_2 are heart rate, myocardial tension and myocardial contractility, and in order to provoke dysfunction due to ischemia, some form of stress is required to increase one or more of these factors.

As the heart can develop only a small oxygen debt, a continuous supply of oxygen is needed in order to maintain contractile activity. Oxygen supply may therefore be the limiting factor for adequate adaptation to any increase in workload [6]. This supply is dependent on coronary blood flow [7], which in the setting of coronary disease is most influenced by the presence of anatomic stenoses. Moreover, ischemia involves not only oxygen deprivation, but also inadequate removal of metabolites due to reduced perfusion, and this differs from hypoxia or anoxia. In the subendocardium [8], the combination of a greater wall stress, a greater resistance to flow and a higher metabolic demand due to a greater degree of shortening results in a lower perfusion rate and a greater susceptibility to ischemia. Other influences, including hydraulic, mechanical, metabolic, neuro-humoral factors, and the oxygen-carrying properties of hemoglobin influence oxygen supply to a lesser degree.

1.1.2 *Pathogenesis of Myocardial Ischemia*

The final common pathway of ischemia is a mismatch between nutrient supply and demand at the level of the cardiac myocyte, and is usually provoked by circumstances necessitating increased nutrient requirements. This situation may arise because of the inability to increase coronary supply due to fixed stenoses in epicardial vessels, reduced coronary supply due to vasoconstriction, and diseases of small vessels.

The commonest mechanism of ischemia is due to reduced coronary blood flow secondary to fixed stenoses. In these circumstances, the severity of stenosis determines the clinical picture. Coronary perfusion at rest is maintained at normal levels until stenoses are severe ($>$ 90% of coronary diameter), at which stage the patient suffers ischemia at rest. Ischemia may be induced by stenoses of lesser severity if they prevent the development of coronary hyperemia in response to increased oxygen demand. This may occur in the presence of stenoses $>$ 50% diameter [9]. However, although stenoses of between 50 and 90% may induce ischemia by reduction of coronary vasodilator reserve, the severity of narrowings and their physiologic effects correlate poorly [10]. Generally, lesser degrees of stenoses require greater amounts of demand (and hence coronary hyperemia) to induce ischemia;

stenoses of 70 to 90% are reliably associated with stress-induced ischemia, whereas those of 50 to 70% may or may not be flow-limiting.

Coronary vasospasm may occur in normal or abnormal vessels. Its occurrence in normal vessels is rare, but accounts for the development of ischemia due solely to reduced blood supply, without increased demand. More commonly, vasomotor tone may modulate the severity of eccentric stenoses, causing variations in exercise capacity from time to time [11].

The importance of small vessel disease in the heart has probably been overstated, and the above mechanisms certainly account for the majority of ischemic episodes. However, small vessel disease may contribute to the development of ischemia in some diseases, principally diabetes [12]. However, the major cause of small vessel disease is probably left ventricular hypertrophy, where vascular compression and inadequate angiogenesis may produce ischemia of hypertrophied myocardium independent of epicardial coronary disease [13].

1.1.3 *Pathophysiology of Myocardial Ischemia*

The various stress tests to detect or assess coronary artery disease reproduce the imbalance between myocardial oxygen demand and supply which precipitate ischemia [14], and this in turn is manifest as impairment of ventricular function. The precise mechanism by which ischemia impairs left ventricular function remains undefined. Ischemia rapidly reduces the rate of ATP usage (within 10 to 15 seconds of its onset), but although this parallels the suppression of contractile function, it may not account for dysfunction because the onset of contractile failure precedes the decline of myocardial ATP content [15]. Contractile failure may be promoted by a slight initial decrease in ATP causing a reduction of influx of Ca^{2+} across the sarcolemma and from the sarcoplasmic reticulum. However, functional changes during ischemia are unlikely to solely reflect a decrease of total intracellular Ca^{2+}, which actually rises during ischemia [16]. Another important mechanism may relate to reduction in the Ca^{2+} sensitivity of the myofilaments, interfering with the ability of Ca^{2+} to modulate the force-generating properties of the contractile proteins. Finally, the high $[H^+]$ induced by ischemia may compete with Ca^{2+} for the troponin receptors, resulting in impairment in the actin-myosin interaction, and failure in contractility.

1.1.4 *Effects of Myocardial Ischemia*

Irrespective of its cause, myocardial ischemia in a single coronary territory is associated with three clinical manifestations: abnormal regional left ventricular function, ECG changes, and angina. The loss of normal contractile activity in that vascular bed rapidly results in asynergy, which is recognizable at echocardiography [17]. Acute coronary occlusion provokes paradoxical motion (systolic bulging or dyskinesis) in the central ischemic zone, reduced contraction (akinesis or hypokinesis) in the adjacent zone and compensatory hyperkinesis in the surrounding unaffected myocardium [18]. Ischemia-induced alterations of systolic function occur very rapidly – during coronary angioplasty, Wijns [19] showed a regional increase in left ventricular stiffness within 20 seconds of coronary occlusion. Indeed, left ventricular distensibility decreases before the onset of systolic failure [20]. The sequence of functional events induced by ischemia begins with diminished left ventricular compliance, followed by decreased myocardial contractility and increased left ventricular end-diastolic pressure. These changes are evidenced at echocardiography by alterations of transmitral flow patterns, abnormal regional systolic function and eventual left ventricular cavity enlargement and reduction of overall left ventricular function.

Models involving coronary occlusion do not equate closely to clinical stress testing, and a closer analogy is based upon gradations of coronary bloodflow reduction. Such experiments have shown a predictable relationship between reductions of flow and function, but for detectable wall motion abnormalities to occur, flow must be reduced to 50% in at least 5% of the myocardium [21].

From the standpoint of the ECG, the genesis of ST segment depression reflects the particular sensitivity of the subendocardium to ischemia. The ischemic myocyte is able to contribute less energy to the Na^+/K^+ pump, resulting in losses of intracellular potassium [22], and partial depolarization of the cells within the ischemic zone. These cells are thus at more negative potential than normal depolarized cells during systole, creating an electric current from the epicardium to the endocardium (ie. away from surface electrodes), resulting in ST depression. While changes in the ST segment and regional dysfunction are therefore both manifestations of ischemia, their time-course may differ, and discrepancies (the presence of one without the other) are not uncommon (see Chapter 5).

The mechanism of the third clinical manifestation – angina pectoris – may be less associated with oxygen supply than the reduction of solute "washout". Acidosis and elevated potassium concentration in the involved tissues may trigger release from the myocardial cells of substances such as adenosine, bradykinin, histamine, or serotonin, to which the sensory intracardiac unmyelinated sympathetic system appear to be extremely sensitive. These mechanisms can be modulated by the endorphine level during stress-induced ischemia [23].

Experimental and clinical experience [24–28] suggests that regional wall motion abnormalities may precede angina or ECG changes. During complete and acute interruption of blood flow during coronary angioplasty, Hauser [27] noted that coronary occlusion was followed by wall motion abnormalities in 86%, 19 ± 8 seconds after balloon inflation; ST segment shifts in 36%, 30 ± 5 seconds after balloon inflation and chest pain in 41%, 39 ± 10 seconds after balloon inflation. In this setting, the "ischemic cascade" [29] describes a pathophysiologic continuum that begins with the abrupt onset of perfusion

Local ischemia

↓

Abnormal diastolic performance

↓

Abnormal regional systolic function

↓

ECG abnormalities

↓

Chest pain

Figure 1.1. Sequence of phenomena induced by ischemia according to the "ischemic cascade" theory.

abnormalities and terminates with the recognized clinical expressions of ischemia (Figure 1.1).

The above studies share the limitation of an experimental design involving "supply-based" ischemia. Their application to the usual clinical setting of "demand-led" ischemia assumes that the timing of these events is equivalent in this situation. Fortunately, both experimental data on graded reductions of flow [30] and clinical experience reassures us that this is so.

1.1.5 *Physiological Basis for Stress-induced Ischemia*

Techniques involving increases in O_2 demand (exercise, pacing or dobutamine stress) or reductions in O_2 supply (vasoactive stress) can both be utilized to demonstrate ischemia in patients with coronary artery disease.

a. Exercise-induced Ischemia. During exercise, the three major determinants of oxygen consumption, heart-rate, blood pressure, and inotropic state all increase with increasing cardiac work. Unless coronary perfusion increases to satisfy the resulting oxygen demand, the myocardium will become ischemic. This relationship is modulated to some extent by other factors, including body position and coronary tone. A change from supine to upright position results in marked blood volume shifts to the legs and abdominal organs, decreasing venous return, left ventricular end-diastolic volume and pressure, stroke volume and cardiac index [31], all of which reduce cardiac work and delay the ischemic threshold [32]. Likewise, dynamic changes in coronary artery tone at the site of atherosclerotic plaques can be induced during exercise, contributing an element of vasospasm.

b. Pacing-induced Ischemia. The primary mechanism for the induction of ischemia during pacing is the development of tachycardia, which exceeds that obtained at pharmacologic stress and may be made equivalent to that of exercise. Augmentations of blood pressure and inotropic state are minor and secondary. There may also be an element of vasospasm; Nabel [33] has shown that a simple increase in heart rate induced by pacing resulted in modest vasodilation in patients with normal coronary arteries, but that coronary stenoses were associated with paradoxical loss in luminal size, suggesting that a reduction in coronary supply may also be involved in increasing heart rate-induced ischemia.

c. Dobutamine-induced Ischemia. The inotropic activity of dobutamine reflects a combination of $alpha_1$ and $beta_1$ stimulation [34], and is equivalent in efficacy to that of epinephrine. In the vasculature, the $alpha_2$ vasodilatory effect of dobutamine is offset by the $beta_1$ vasoconstrictor activity, thus limiting the net changes in blood pressure following dobutamine infusion and producing a potential limitation to the test due to the development of hypotension. Thus, although the inotropic state is enhanced by this drug, the more important determinants of myocardial oxygen consumption (heart-rate and blood pressure) are augmented to a lesser extent than is possible using submaximal exercise. Nonetheless, the development of an ischemic response in presence of coronary stenoses is analogous to that witnessed with exercise – with initially a reduction of the positive inotropic effect [35] and then regional ventricular dysfunction.

While the development of ischemia appears to correlate mainly with the chronotropic effects of this drug [36], the degree of ischemia may outstrip that expected at the attained level of cardiac work, possibly due to metabolic effects known of as "oxygen-wasting". This has been suggested by an augmentation of the ratio between MVO_2 and the pressure-volume area (defined as the sum of the external mechanical work and the end-systolic elastic potential energy) during infusion of catecholamines (especially dobutamine), despite independence from heart-rate changes [37–41]. Similarly, a recent comparison of cardiac workload at the time of onset of regional wall motion abnormalities during dobutamine and exercise stress found dyskinesia to occur at significantly lower rate-pressure product during dobutamine stress, suggesting the involvement of other mechanisms than simply an increase in external cardiac work [42]. The cause of this "oxygen-wasting" is unclear, but could reflect an increased energy cost of excitation-contraction coupling and Ca^{2+} reuptake after adrenergic stimulation [43].

d. Vasodilator-induced Ischemia. The coronary vasodilators induce myocardial ischemia by a paradoxical impairment of oxygen supply. These agents exert their effects through the reduction of collateral flow due to lowering of pressure in supplying vessels. This "steal" process may be "vertical" (redirection from the endocardium to the epicardium), "horizontal" (redirection from areas supplied by a stenosed artery to normally perfused areas), or involve other mechanisms including the passive collapse of stenoses, systemic steal (reducing coronary flow due to reduced perfusion pressure) and luxury perfusion [44]. In addition, a degree of increased demand may contribute to the genesis of ischemia.

The major coronary vasodilators used for stress echocardiography are adenosine and dipyridamole. Adenosine is a very potent endogenous vasodilator, which may be administered directly or indirectly (via dipyridamole). Dipyridamole blocks the cellular uptake of adenosine, leading to an increased concentration of adenosine in both the myocardial and the arterial wall [45]. They will be discussed further in Chapter 5.

e. Vasoconstrictor-induced Ischemia. Coronary spasm may be a contributor to the development of myocardial ischemia, but is uncommonly its only cause. The mechanism of coronary vasomotion is not well understood, and the vasoconstrictor stressors (hyperventilation or ergonovine) may well not be representative of the underlying pathophysiology. These tests are not commonly indicated, but are discussed further in Chapter 5.

There is, therefore, a perplexing choice of exercise, pacing and pharmacologic stress agents for use with stress echocardiography. On the basis of current evidence, no single stress technique appears to enjoy unqualified superiority, and the selection of a stress must be tailored to the clinical question being addressed in each individual patient. These issues will be discussed further in Chapters 3, 4 and 5.

1.2 Detection of Ischemic Dyssynergy with Echocardiography

1.2.1 *M-mode Echocardiography*

M-mode echocardiography has the advantage of a high sampling rate and provides accurate spatial and temporal measurements. This technique has been used for the identification of myocardial ischemia [46]. However, it is an approach with important limitations. The M-mode beam interrogates only an "ice-pick" view of the heart, and even with tedious mapping, not all of the ventricle may be visible. Moreover, the strengths of the methodology apply only to when a view perpendicular to the chamber is available; off-axis measurements may be misleading. Thus, stress M-mode echocardiography is not attractive for routine clinical application, though it may be a useful adjunct to two-dimensional imaging (see Chapter 2).

1.2.2 *Two-dimensional Echocardiography*

The spatial orientation and real-time imaging provided by two-dimensional echocardiography are ideal for the purpose of identifying myocardial ischemia [47]. Stress two-dimensional echocardiography has been attempted since the late 1970's [48]. However, the growth of stress echocardiography as a clinical tool has been a later development, which has largely paralleled the development of digital image processing [49]. Following the establishment of its diagnostic role, stress echocardiography has progressed to further applications, including the identification of viable myocardium and evaluation of the efficacy of therapy.

The disadvantages of two-dimensional echocardiography for imaging the response of the heart to stress relate to issues of subjectiveness and image quality. Four other investigations are available to give a two-dimensional assessment of left ventricular function; nuclear scintigraphy (including first pass, and gated planar and SPECT imaging), contrast ventriculography, computed tomography, and magnetic resonance imaging. While attempts have been made to perform stress imaging with each, the last three are currently either too invasive or too expensive to be attractive for clinical purposes. The comparison between echocardiography and nuclear ventriculography will be discussed in Chapter 7.

In conclusion, while stress 2D echocardiography is being used on a routine clinical basis in some centers, its broader dispersion has been limited, in part, by the concentration of expertise in relatively few institutions. The subsequent chapters are aimed at dispelling some misconceptions about the difficulty and accuracy of the technique, and address practical issues pertaining to the performance of the test, including the definition of optimal stressors. The book also seeks to define the place of the stress echocardiogram in the context of the other non-invasive techniques for the diagnosis of ischemia.

References

1. Gibbons WR, Zygmunt AC. Excitation-contraction coupling in the heart. In: Fozzard HA, editor. The heart and cardiovascular system. 2nd ed. New York: Raven Press, 1991.
2. Ford LE. Mechanical manifestations of activation in cardiac muscle. Circ Res 1991;68:621–35.
3. Gwathmey JK, Hajjar RJ. Relation between steady-state force and intracellular [Ca^+] in intact human myocardium: Index of myofibrillar responsiveness to Ca^+. Circulation 1990;82:1266–78.
4. Katz AM. Physiology of the heart. New York: Raven Press, 1977.
5. Heineman FW, Balaban RS. Control of myocardial oxygen consumption by work. In: Fozzard HA, editor. The heart and cardiovascular system. 2nd ed. New York: Raven Press, 1991.
6. Ardehali A, Ports TA. Myocardial oxygen supply and demand. Chest 1990;98:699–705.
7. Young MA, Vatner SF. Regulation of large coronary artery. Circ Res 1986;59:579–96.

8. Bell JR, Fox AC. Pathogenesis of subendocardial ischemia. Am J Med Sci 1974;268:2–11.
9. Gould KL, Schelbert HR, Phelps ME, Hoffman EJ. Non-invasive assessment of coronary stenoses with myocardial perfusion imaging during pharmacologic coronary vasodilation. V. Detection of 47 percent coronary diameter stenosis with intravenous nitrogen-13 ammonia and emission computed tomography in intact dogs. Am J Cardiol 1979;43:200–8.
10. White CW, Wright CB, Doty DB *et al.* Does visual interpretation of the coronary arteriogram predict the physiologic significance of a coronary stenosis? N Engl J Med 1984;310:819–24.
11. Gorlin R, Fuster V, Ambrose JA. Anatomic-physiologic links between acute coronary syndromes. Circulation 1986;74:6–12.
12. Van Hoeven KH, Factor SM. The diabetic heart: Clinical, experimental and pathological features. Acta Cardiol 1991;46:329–39.
13. O'Gorman DJ, Sheridan DJ. Abnormalities of the coronary circulation associated with left ventricular hypertrophy. Clin Sci 1991;81:703–13.
14. Braunwald E, Sobel BE. Coronary blood flow and myocardial ischemia. In Braunwald E, editor. Heart disease. 4th ed. Philadelphia: Saunders, 1992.
15. Kanaide H, Yoshimura R, Makino N, Nakamura M. Regional myocardial function and metabolism during acute coronary artery occlusion. Am J Physiol 1982;242:H980–9.
16. Kihara Y, Grossman W, Morgan JP. Direct measurements of changes in intracellullar calcium transients during hypoxia, ischemia, and reperfusion of the intact mammalian heart. Circ Res 1989;65:1029–44.
17. Kerber RE, Marcus ML, Erhardt J, Wilson R, Abboud FM. Correlation between echocardiographically-demonstrated segmental dyskinesis and regional myocardial perfusion. Circulation 1975;52:1097–103.
18. Lew WYW, Chen Z, Guth B, Covell JW. Mechanisms of augmented segment shortening in nonischemic areas during acute ischemia of the canine left ventricle. Circ Res 1985;56:351–8.
19. Wijns W, Serruys PW, Slager CJ *et al.* Effects of coronary occlusion during percutaneous transluminal angioplasty in humans on left ventricular chamber stiffness and regional diastolic pressure-radius relations. J Am Coll Cardiol 1986;7:455–63.
20. Aroesty JM, McKay RG, Heller GV *et al.* Simultaneous assessment of left ventricular systolic and diastolic dysfunction during pacing-induced ischemia. Circulation 1985;71:889–900.
21. Armstrong WF. Echocardiography in coronary artery disease. Progr Cardiovasc Dis 1988;30:267–88.
22. Morena H, Janse MJ, Fiolet JWT, Krieger WJG, Crijns H, Durrer D. Comparison of the effects of regional ischemia, hypoxia, hyperkalemia, and acidosis on intracellular and extracellular potentials and metabolism in the isolated porcine heart. Circ Res 1980;46:634–46.
23. Sheps DS, Adams KF, Hindliter A *et al.* Endorphins are related to pain perception in coronary artery disease. Am J Cardiol 1987;59:523–7.
24. Battler A, Froelicher VF, Gallagher KP *et al.* Dissociation between regional myocardial dysfunction and ECG changes during ischemia in the conscious dog. Circulation 1980;62:735–44.
25. Gallagher KP, Matsuzaki M, Osakada G *et al.* Effect of exercise on the relationship between myocardial blood flow and systolic wall thickening in dogs with acute coronary stenosis. Circ Res 1983;52:716–29.
26. Sugishita Y, Koseki S, Matsuda M *et al.* Dissociation between regional myocardial dysfunction and ECG changes during myocardial ischemia in patients with angina pectoris. Am Heart J 1983;106:1–8.
27. Hauser AM, Vellappillil G, Ramos RG *et al.* Sequence of mechanical, electrocardiographical and clinical effects of repeated coronary artery occlusion in human beings: echocardiographic observations during coronary angioplasty. J Am Coll Cardiol 1985;5:193–7.
28. Wohlgelernter D, Cleman M, Highman HA *et al.* Regional myocardial dysfunction during

coronary angioplasty: evaluation by two-dimensinnal echocardiography and 12–lead electrocardiography. J Am Coll Cardiol 1986;7:1245–54.
29. Nesto RW, Kowalchuck GJ. The ischemic cascade: Temporal sequence of hemodynamic, electrocardiographic and symptomatic expressions of ischemia. Am J Cardiol 1987;57:23C–27C.
30. Wyatt HL, Forrester JS, Tyberg JV *et al.* Effect of graded reductions in regional coronary perfusion on regional and total cardiac function. Am J Cardiol 1975;36:185–92.
31. Flamm SD, Taki J, Moore R *et al.* Redistribution of regional and organ blood volume and effect on cardiac function in relation to upright exercise intensity in healthy human subjects. Circulation 1990;81:1550–9.
32. Froelicher VF. Exercise and the heart. Clinical concepts. 2nd ed. Chicago: Year Book Medical Publishers Inc, 1987.
33. Nabel EG, Selwyn AP, Ganz P. Paradoxical narrowing of atherosclerotic coronary arteries induced by increase in heart rate. Circulation 1990; 81:850–9.
34. Ruffolo RR. The pharmacology of dobutamine. Am J Med Sci 1987;294:244–8.
35. McGillem MJ, DeBoe SF, Friedman HZ, Mancini GBJ. The effect of dopamine and dobutamine on regional function in the presence of rigid coronary stenoses and subcritical impairments of reactive hyperemia. Am Heart J 1988;115:970–7.
36. Rude RE, Izquierdo C, Buja LM, Willerson JT. Effects of inotropic and chronotropic stimuli on acute myocardial ischemic injury. Studies with dobutamine in the anestetized dog. Circulation 1982;1321–8.
37. Suga H, Hisano R, Goto Y, Yamada O, Igarashi Y. Effect of positive inotropic agents on the relation between oxygen consumption and systolic pressure volume area in canine left ventricule. Circ Res 1983;53:306–18.
38. Suga H, Futaki S, Tanaka N *et al.* Paired pulse pacing increases cardiac O_2 consumption for activation without changing efficiency of contractile machinery in canine left ventricle. Heart Vessels 1988;4:79–87.
39. Vasu MA, O'Keefe DD, Kapellakis GZ *et al.* Myocardial oxygen consumption: effects of epinephrine, isoproterenol, dopamine, norepinephrine and dobutamine. Am J Physiol 1978;235:H237–41.
40. Vanoverschelde J-L, Wijns W, Essamri B *et al.* Do cathecholamines cause oxygen-wasting in the normal human left ventricle? [abstract] Circulation 1992;86:I–247.
41. Mairesse GH, D'Hondt AM, Vanoverschelde JL *et al.* Are dobutamine-induced wall motion abnormalities only caused by increased cardiac work ? [abstract] Echocardiography 1993 (in press).
42. Ohgoshi Y, Goto Y, Futaki S, Yaku H, Suga H. Sensitivities of cardiac O_2 consumption and contractility to catecholamines in dogs. Am J Physiol 1991;261:H196–205.
43. Chung N, Wu X, Ritman EL. Left ventricular oxygen consumption and pressure-volume area: the role of norepinephrine and verapamil. Am J Physiol 1991;261:H77–82.
44. Picano E. Dipyridamole-echocardiography test: historical background and physiological basis. Eur Heart J 1989;10:365–76.
45. Moser GH, Schrader J, Deussen A. Turnover of adenosine in plasma of human and dog blood. Am J Physiol 1989;256:C799–806.
46. Mason SJ, Weiss JL, Weisfeldt ML, Garrison JB, Fortuin NJ. Exercise echocardiography: Detection of wall motion abnormalities during ischemia. Circulation 1979;59:50–4.
47. Kerber RE, Marcus ML, Abboud FM. Echocardiography in experimentally induced myocardial ischemia. Am J Med 1977;63:21.
48. Wann LS, Faris JB, Childress RH, Dillon JC, Weyman AE, Feigenbaum H. Exercise cross-sectional echocardiography in ischemic heart disease. Circulation 1979;60:1300–6.
49. West SR, Feigenbaum H, Armstrong WF, Green D, Dillon JC. Split-screen simultaneous digital imaging of rest and stress echocardiogram – A new method for evaluation of exercise induced wall motion abnormalities [abstract]. J Am Coll Cardiol 1984;3:563.

2. How to Perform Stress Echocardiography – Practical Aspects

Regional left ventricular systolic function is impaired by myocardial ischemia, and the extent and severity of ischemia determine the time-course and spatial distribution of these abnormalities. The principle of stress echocardiography is to image the heart at rest, and to compare these images with those obtained following stress, with the implication that deterioration in regional function corresponds to the presence of ischemia. The ability of echocardiography to record the severity of regional dysfunction, as well as its spatial extent and temporal distribution, permits an appreciation of the severity of coronary pathology as well as its presence or absence. As exercise-induced ischemia is usually transient, the most reliable data are generally acquired at peak stress or (if peak images are not feasible) within the shortest possible time after exercise [1]. Moreover, the induced wall motion abnormality may be subtle if the stenosis is moderate, situated distally, or if the patient is stressed submaximally. These considerations dictate that stress echocardiograms need to be not only acquired rapidly, but should be of the highest quality as well. The successful performance of stress echocardiography is therefore based upon meticulous attention to practical detail.

2.1 Equipment for Stress Echocardiography

2.1.1 *Echocardiograph Devices*

The technical difficulties of stress echocardiography necessitate use of the best available echocardiography equipment for this purpose [2]. Devices more than 5 years old are noticeably inferior to current models and probably should not be used for stress echocardiography. Recent advances in computing have permitted larger numbers of transducer crystals and improved signal processing, with a commensurate improvement in two-dimensional image quality. The development of relatively small transducers has also facilitated rapid post-exercise imaging. However, as with resting echocardiography, the selection between currently available echocardiography machines is one based upon personal preference, familiarity and cost.

While most patients with suspected coronary disease are readily studied

T.H. Marwick, Stress Echocardiography, 11–37.

by echocardiography, the prevalence of smoking and obesity in this population means that the superior penetration of a 2.5 MHz transducer is usually needed to visualize the deeper regions of the heart, even if this is at the cost of some spatial resolution [3]. As with all two-dimensional echocardiography, time should be taken to optimize images in each individual patient. In particular, excessive gain settings should be avoided, as this may obscure endocardial detail. Finally, depth must be altered to optimize image size, definition and frame-rate (which falls with increasing depth).

2.1.2 *Image Processing for Stress Echocardiography*

i) *Conventional Recording Methods*. The strength of two dimensional echocardiography is the ability to see the moving heart; data recording therefore requires a medium offering continuous visualization of images. Until recently, this has necessitated the use of video-tape, but video recordings have several disadvantages for stress echocardiography. First, there is some degradation of image quality in the course of recording and playing back from tape – this may assume importance with respect to defining the endocardium, especially if this is ill-defined due to suboptimal image quality. Second, freeze-frame images (and those scanned slowly) may be impaired by artifacts (though this is less of a problem with modern Super-VHS systems). Most importantly, video playback is literally "real-time", so that comparison of regional wall motion before and after exercise requires the interpreter to remember pre-test function in each individual segment when the post-exercise images are reviewed. In effect, this mandates much playing and rewinding of the video tape to facilitate comparisons between images. This process is time-consuming and does not lend itself readily to communication with non-cardiologists, nor indeed, non-echocardiographers.

ii) *Image Digitization*. Recent advances in computing have made digital recording a practical alternative to the conventional, video recording method. Although some "all-digital" systems are available, generally, this method usually requires digitization of video images (derived from the echocardiography machine or a videotape player), by a "frame-grabber" incorporated in a modified personal computer. This process may be performed after the stress ("off-line"), permitting selection of a specific cardiac cycle. However, this is time-consuming, and most centers now perform direct ("on-line") digitization from the echocardiograph, which is less tedious. The on-line approach also avoids image degradation inherent in recording onto, and reading back from video-tape, and is readily incorporated into the imaging protocol. For these reasons, most busy clinical laboratories use this online processing. On-line acquisition may be possible using echocardiography devices having combined digitizing capacity; these are convenient and economic on space requirements, but have the disadvantage that the acquisition device is required in order to report the studies – a problem which may be avoided with separate digitizing equipment. Finally, a clear distinction should be made between digitizing devices and the digital cine-loop facility built into most modern echocardiography machines. The latter are restricted by limited memory, although the incorporation of optical disks has improved their ability to archive data in digital format.

The digitization process involves division of an image into a frame comprising a grid of pixels, each containing data corresponding to the signal amplitude (gray scale) at that site. There exists a difficult balance between the benefits of a large quantity of pixels (high spatial resolution) and/or a large number of gray levels (good contrast resolution), and the disadvantages of extensive processing time and the storage of voluminous amounts of data. The amount of data stored in each frame reflects the resolution employed – this varies from 65,536 kilobytes using 256 × 256 pixel resolution, to 262,144 with 512 × 512 pixel resolution. Decisions regarding the sampling density are best based upon the inherent resolution of the echocardiographic image, which is of the order of 1 to 1.5 mm in the axial dimension, and less in lateral and cross-plane dimension [4]. For images acquired at a depth of 18 cm, a 256 × 256 matrix is appropriate, as this gives each pixel an axial dimension of 0.7 mm, or about half of the inherent resolution of the system.

Data processing requirements are also dictated by the number of frames of interest. Digitization of every video frame of the cardiac cycle at a heart-rate of 60/minute (ie one second per beat) at a frame-rate of 30/second, would require 30 frames – or nearly 2 megabytes of memory using a 256 × 256 matrix. Even with larger memory available in current computers, such amounts of data are unwieldy. There is therefore some need to be selective about the number of frames acquired. Fortunately, the systolic component of the cardiac cycle is of most importance for stress echocardiography, so that using an interim delay (interval between frames) of 40 to 60 msec, 8 frames (over 280 to 420 msec) can readily form a systolic cine-loop at most physiologic heart-rates (Figure 2.1). In order to examine systole, the sequence is initiated (following a "start-delay"), by the R-wave of the electrocardiogram, either through an external signal (R-wave beep), or through scanning the scrolling ECG incorporated in the video image. Generally, to minimize ECG artifacts post-exercise, it is better to use a signal exported from the treadmill ECG device than one derived from the echocardiograph, which may also be delayed by the process of updating the video image [5]. Use of a 256 × 256 resolution with an 8–frame cine-loop requires only about 1/2 megabyte per cine-loop, which may be further compressed for storage. Digital storage can be performed using floppy discs (which carry a risk of degradation as well as being relatively expensive both in cost and storage space), a hard disk (though this has limited volume and is unfavorable for long term storage), or optical disks (which have a larger storage capacity and will probably become the best choice).

Image digitization brings with it both benefits and disadvantages. The former pertain to both acquisition and interpretation. Image quality may be

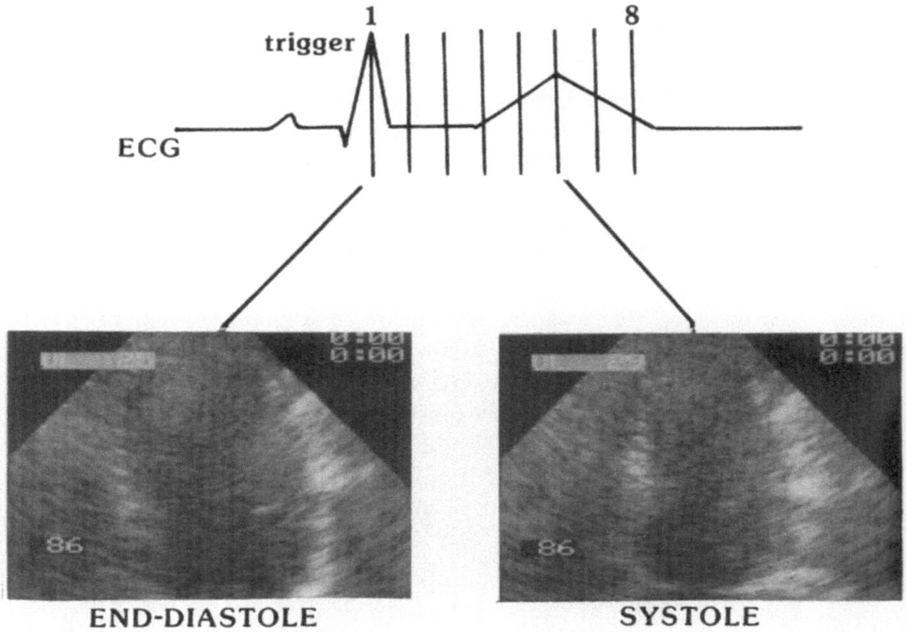

Figure 2.1. Principle of systolic triggering for formation of a cine-loop. The first image (end-diastole) follows the electrocardiographic R-wave (after a "start delay"), with subsequent frames separated by an "interim delay".

enhanced by avoidance of video-tape storage (especially if the data are digitized on-line), and digital images have a linear increment of gray-scale. Image acquisition (especially during and after stress) may be facilitated by on-line digitization, as sequential cine-loops may be rapidly viewed to ensure that an image of adequate quality has been acquired before moving on to the next view in the shortest possible time. The cine-loop facilitates image interpretation by allowing the observer to compare the same wall segments in a side-by-side rest-stress format. It also enables integration of cardiac motion both temporally and spatially, thus minimizing the effects of body and respiratory movement. Image interpretation is also enhanced by the ability to play cine-loops side-by-side. Individual frames are readily reviewed, so that specific attention may be paid to the first half of systole (which limits the influence of translational movement) in the interpretation of the study. Finally, this technology has benefits for reviewing any type of echocardiographic data rapidly and in condensed form. A sequence of several studies (eg during the course of myocardial infarction, or before and after intervention) may be "re-mixed" digitally, enabling responses at temporally separate resting or exercise examinations to be reviewed side-by-side (Figure 2.2).

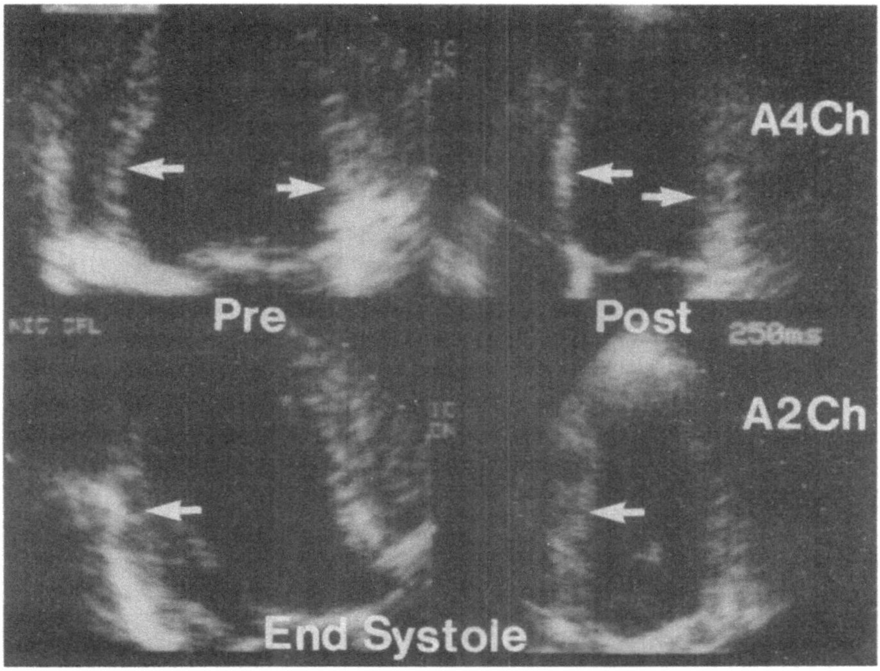

Figure 2.2. Side-by-side comparison of resting end-systolic apical 4-chamber (A4Ch) and apical 2-chamber (A2Ch) images before and after revascularization. The inferior, lateral and septal walls are seen to be akinetic initially, with improvement after revascularization (arrows). Reproduced with permission of the American Journal of Cardiology.

Although serial studies may be reviewed on video tape, the time required to find, review and compare them limits the feasibility of this activity.

The disadvantages of image digitization pertain mainly to problems related to selection of the data to be digitized. As the method involves comparison of single cardiac cycles, these must be of the same regions of myocardium (hence the window and view must be the same), and care must be taken to avoid sampling extrasystolic cycles. The timing of the cycle is also crucial, and errors in triggering may make the digital cine-loops useless. Finally, technical problems with the digitizer or corruption of the archived data risk loss of the study. All of these reasons mandate duplicate recording of all studies on video tape, which should be reviewed if the diagnosis is uncertain.

The balance between the advantages and disadvantages of image digitization is best addressed by a comparison of interpretations using the two techniques in the same patients. Such data are scarce; in our own experience of comparing the findings in 86 patients [6], the accuracies of both dobutamine and exercise echocardiograms (64% and 85%) were enhanced by digital processing, compared with interpretation from video tape (with which accuracies were 55% and 77%, respectively). For both dobutamine and exercise studies, this benefit occurred mainly through a small improvement in sensitivity, at comparable levels of specificity. However, the numbers involved were not large enough for these differences to attain statistical significance. Our own practice is to employ on-line digitization for all studies, as we believe that the process facilitates and shortens interpretation and enhances the ability to detect mild ischemia.

2.2 Acquisition of Stress Echocardiograms

2.2.1 *Stress Protocols for Combination with Echocardiography*

In a fashion analogous to scintigraphic approaches, stress echocardiography may be performed with exercise and non-exercise stresses. In general, preparations for stress testing are little influenced by the addition of echocardiography. Unlike the scintigraphic approaches, unless pharmacologic stress is to be used, an intravenous line is not required. Some logistic details do require attention, however. If exercise stress is selected, the examination bed should be positioned close to the treadmill or bicycle, to facilitate rapid acquisition of post-stress images. A "cut-away" bed (with an indentation under the left chest) may enable easier access to the apical window. Electrocardiographic electrodes may need to be repositioned in order to optimize echocardiographic windows, though this usually involves only leads V2 (left parasternal) and V5 (apical) electrodes. As displacement of the ECG leads may interfere with Q-wave interpretation of the pre-test ECG [7], this adjustment should only be made after the routine resting ECG has been completed. The displacement of the relevant leads (usually by one intercostal space) has a minimal effect on ST-segment interpretation. Finally, the echocardiographic study should not influence the type or performance of the stress protocol, which should be tailored to each patient.

Either treadmill or bicycle exercise may be combined with echocardiography. Pre- and post-treadmill protocols are technically easier, as the patient is supine and relatively immobile. However, imaging is difficult during treadmill stress [8], so the test cannot identify the time of onset of ischemia, which may be a useful index of the physiologic severity of coronary disease. Bicycle stress permits peak exercise imaging, and so may avoid false negative results caused by the rapid resolution of ischemia. These aspects are discussed further in Chapter 3.

For those patients who are unable to perform lower limb exercise, there exist pharmacologic and non-pharmacologic methods for provoking myocardial ischemia. The choices for pharmacologic stress (exercise simulating and vasoactive agents) are discussed in Chapter 4. Other non-exercise approaches include handgrip, cold pressor and pacing stresses [9–12]. Handgrip stress is ineffective, and the cold pressor test is uncomfortable and poorly tolerated.

Transvenous pacing stress is unacceptably invasive, though pacing may be accomplished via the esophagus [11]. Recently, pacing has been performed using electrodes attached to a transesophageal echocardiography probe [12]; because of better contact with the esophagus, this approach has required lower stimulation thresholds and hence less discomfort than the former "pill" electrode. Echocardiographic images are recorded at the end of each stage in a fashion analogous to the approach for pharmacologic stress (Chapter 4).

2.2.2 *Two-dimensional Imaging for Stress Echocardiography*

The performance of stress two-dimensional echocardiography differs only in detail from that of routine echocardiography. Indeed, one of the attractions of using a stress-imaging technique with such excellent resolution of cardiac structure is that nonspecific cardiac symptoms such as chest discomfort atypical for ischemia, and exertional dyspnea may be elucidated. Non-ischemic causes of these symptoms include pericardial disease, pulmonary emboli, aortic and mitral valve disease and cardiac masses. Thus, although some curtailment of the complete echo-Doppler examination is often dictated by the performance of the test in the context of the exercise laboratory, we believe that a brief M-mode and color examination is mandatory at the pre-stress imaging. Patients with significant non-ischemic pathology may then proceed to a more complete study if required.

For stress echocardiography, it is useful to modify the views to attend more to the myocardium than to the valves (for example, long axis parasternal images are often portrayed more vertically than usual). Irrespective of such minor variations, images should comprise apical, parasternal and/or subcostal views [13] before, during (if possible) and after stress. The need to acquire multiple views simply reflects the fact that any small incremental piece of data may facilitate or corroborate a difficult interpretation. Because of the potentially rapid resolution of ischemia, there is also a balance between imaging perfection and speed of acquisition, especially for the post-stress images, where a complete set of imperfect but "readable" images in the first minute may prove more useful than perfect views obtained over several minutes. However, this does not negate the importance of optimizing endocardial definition and avoidance of foreshortening the left ventricular cavity. To assist with the rapid acquisition of on-axis views, some authorities recommend marking the location of the echocardiographic windows, though the utility of this may be limited by movement of the window during or after stress.

The parasternal views offer the optimal geometry between the transducer and the walls of the heart, and hence the best image quality, provided that the echocardiographic window is adequate (Figure 2.3). Images may be enhanced by asking the patient to exhale, and improving the contact between the heart and chest wall by lying as far as possible onto the left side (for supine imaging) or by leaning forward on the bicycle (for upright imaging).

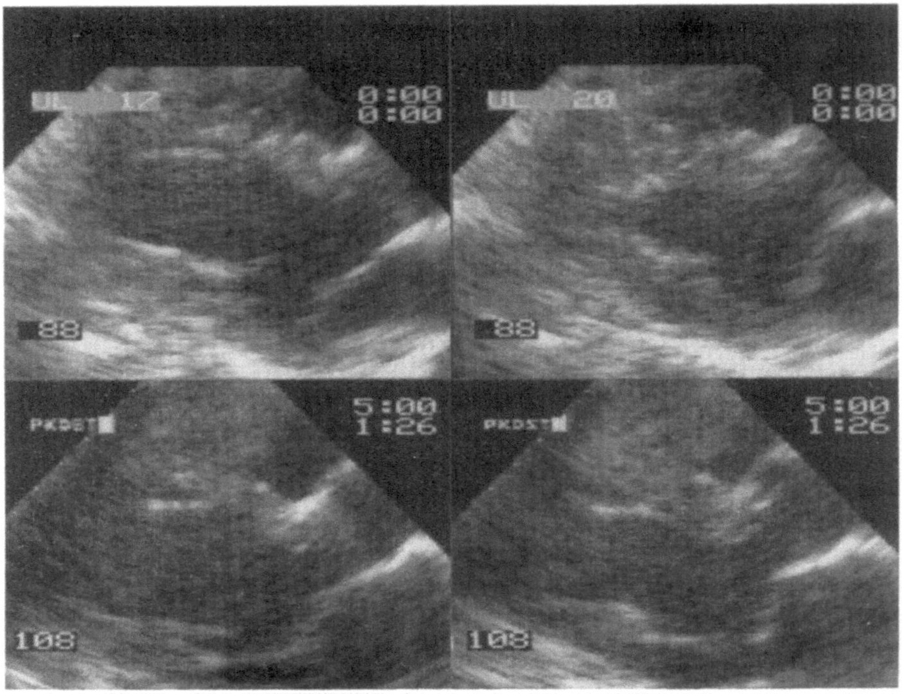

Figure 2.3. Freeze-frame images and traced outlines of the parasternal long axis view of the left ventricle. There is normal resting function (R), with reduction of anteroseptal and posterior

Pictures of good quality may enable wall thickening to be used for interpretation in addition to endocardial excursion. If uncertainty exists about the diagnosis of ischemia in the anteroseptal or posterior walls, the orientation of these walls usually enables M-mode imaging to be used in the identification of delayed contraction.

The other parasternal images are acquired in the short-axis view, which is most commonly acquired at the mid-ventricular (papillary muscle) level. Apical short axis views may be useful to corroborate abnormalities detected in the apical images, but are often technically difficult. Care should be exercised in the performance and interpretation of high (subvalvular) images; although the basal inferior segment (supplied by the posterior descending branch of the right coronary artery) may be well seen in this view, incorporation of the valve plane or even the atrial wall may be misleading. Similarly, tangential cuts may be obtained in any short-axis view, so that the observer should be particularly vigilant for the presence of artifacts. This is not to say that the short axis view should be ignored: if the apical window is of poor quality, the right coronary artery territory (inferior wall) may only be apparent in this view. Moreover, if good quality images are available, they have

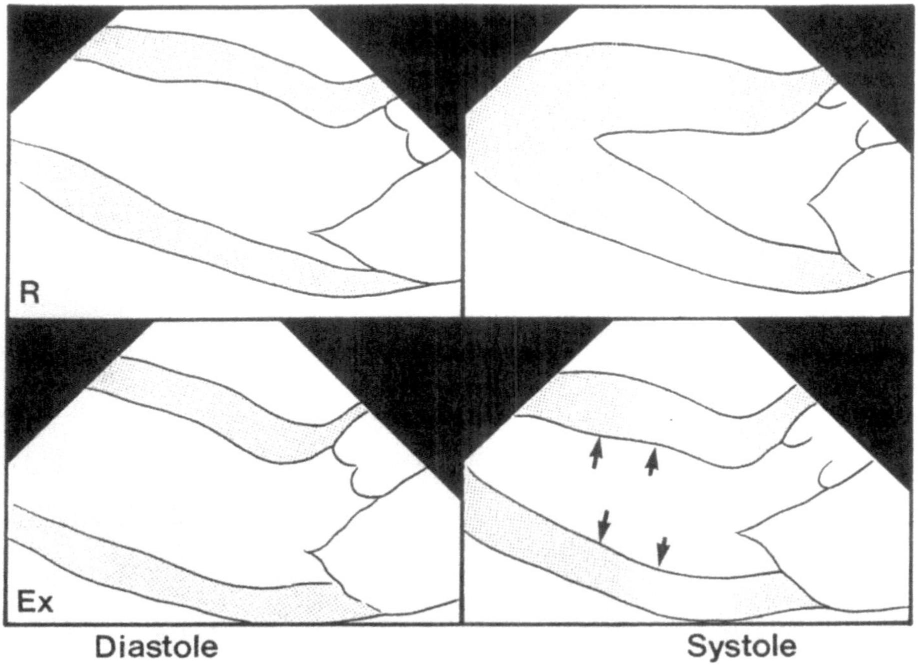

wall excursion and thickening (arrows) after bicycle exercise (Ex), consistent with ischemia of both walls.

been considered by some authors to present the optimal views for visualization of ischemia-induced alterations of ventricular volumes or ejection fraction, although such alterations may be nonspecific for coronary disease. (Figure 2.4).

The availability of apical views is mandatory for obtaining reliable stress echocardiograms. The apex is the most common site of a wall motion abnormality (because it is in the most distal perfusion zone of each coronary artery), and this region is usually not visualized from the parasternal views. Imaging should again concentrate on the myocardium rather than the valves and aorta – this aspect influences the field depth and focusing, and particularly the location of the zoom window for cine-loop acquisition. Some maneuvering may be required to optimize images; if the window is poor, the patient may need to exhale – although sometimes the window is improved by partial inspiration. Finally, the acquisition of a true apical 2–chamber view is required rather than an apical long-axis view (Figure 2.5). This is because the former examines the anterior and inferior walls, while the latter visualizes the antero-septal and posterior walls, thereby duplicating the parasternal long-axis view and neglecting to visualize the territory of the right

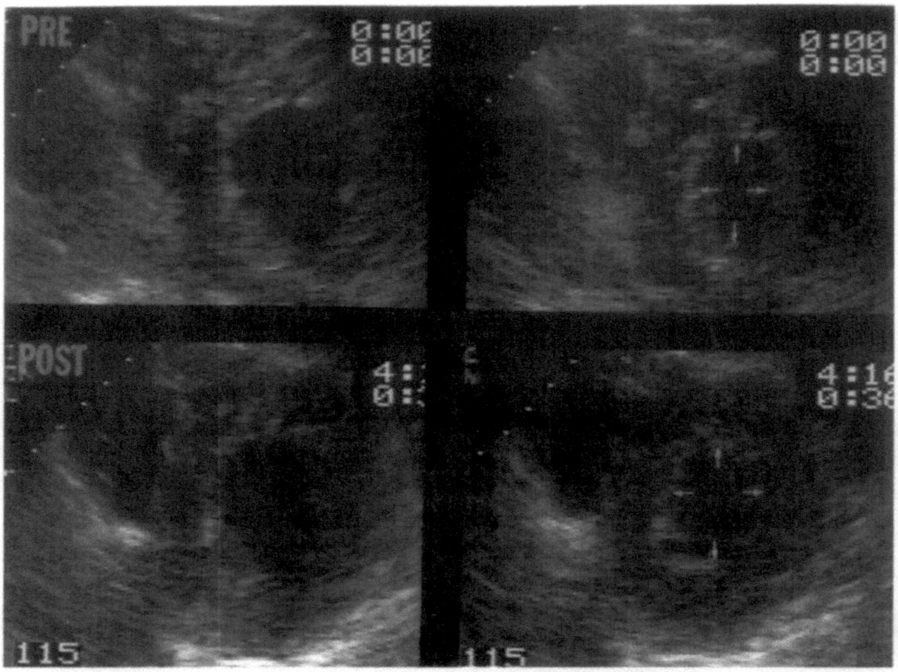

Figure 2.4. Short axis views of the left ventricle in diastole (left) and systole, in a patient without significant coronary disease, before (pre) and after (post) treadmill exercise, showing systolic cavity dilation. Reproduced with permission of the American Journal of Cardiac Imaging.

coronary artery. On the other hand, the apical long-axis view may be used in lieu of the parasternal long-axis if the latter window is poor.

Subcostal views are often not of very good quality at supine imaging. However, during upright imaging, the diaphragm and heart are lower, and closer to the subcostal window, providing potentially useful images. While we do not use these views routinely at upright bicycle echocardiography, they are useful if other views are unsatisfactory. Subcostal views have the advantage of offering the optimal orientation between the ultrasound beam and the endocardium, and have been used for quantitative echocardiography [2]. Used in isolation, however, they do have limitations with respect to permitting a full tomographic evaluation of the ventricle.

There are no firm rules in respect of the imaging sequence for stress echocardiography. Digitizing devices generally label successive views as parasternal long- and short-axis, and apical 4– and 2–chamber in that order; it is therefore convenient to follow this pattern. However, because early post-stress imaging time is particularly valuable, we perform apical views first if the parasternal window is poor, or if resting dysfunction has already identified

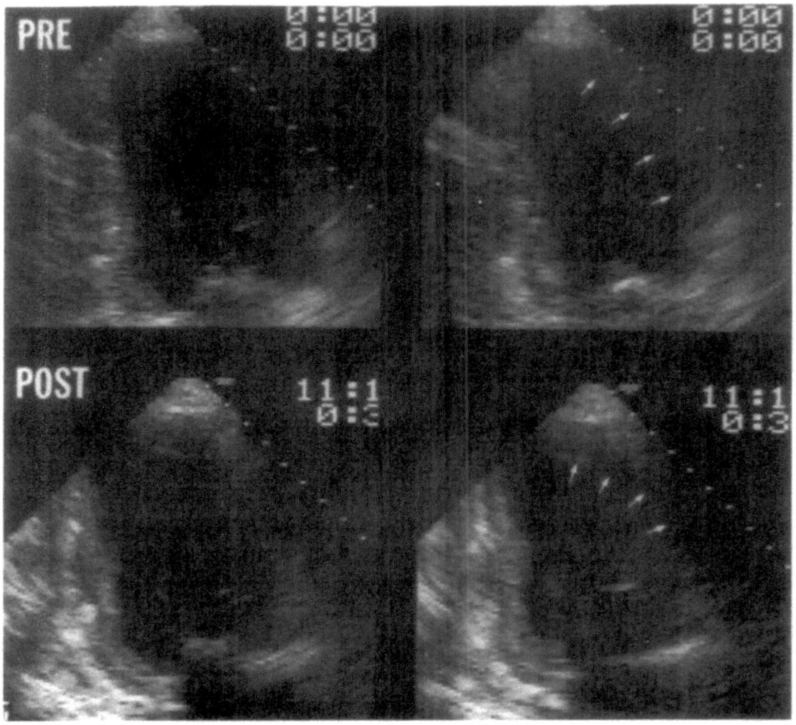

Figure 2.5. Stop-frame images of apical 2-chamber views in a patient with apical anterior wall ischemia (arrows). The aortic valve is not visualized – hence the walls are anterior and inferior, rather than anteroseptal and posterior (compare with Figure 2.3).

wall motion abnormalities in the parasternal view. Finally, while the quality of the echocardiographic images is obviously important, very few patients are unsuitable for this test because of poor image quality. Paradoxically, imaging often improves after stress, so that imperfect resting images should not lead to cancellation of the test.

2.2.3 *Transesophageal Stress Echocardiography*

Without doubt, the greatest limitation to the widespread acceptance of stress echocardiography has been the image quality of standard two-dimensional images. Use of the transesophageal "window" offers enhanced image quality because it avoids problems related to soft tissue attenuation of the ultrasound beam, and permits the use of higher frequency probes [14]. New echocardiographic applications, including tissue characterization and three-dimensional reconstruction, are being studied with this technique, and may be of use in the field of stress echocardiography.

However, despite its benefits in relation to image quality, transesophageal stress echocardiography has not been widely adopted. Initially, the new technique was not routinely applied for the purpose of stress echocardiography because the original transverse plane transesophageal probes offered limited views of the left ventricle (principally, short axis and 4–chamber equivalent). Some difficulties in obtaining reliable apical imaging have remained after the introduction of biplane probes (this limitation being of some importance as the apex is the earliest and most common site of ischemia), but the availability of multiplane imaging has enabled visualization of the entire left ventricle. Recently, the introduction of transesophageal pacing stress (see Chapter 4) has given further impetus to the development of stress transoesophageal echocardiography.Further advances are likely to come in the form of probe miniaturization. However, at present, the procedure is unpleasant for the patient, and seems unlikely to widely replace transthoracic imaging, although some specific indications for it are likely to be found.

2.2.4 *Stress Doppler Studies*

While 2D-echocardiography examines regional wall morphology and function, Doppler studies examine the hemodynamic sequelae of these contractions. Hemodynamic alterations due to ischemia may be reflected in disturbances of either systolic or diastolic flow.

Using a non-imaging Doppler transducer from the suprasternal window, peak aortic bloodflow velocity and acceleration may be obtained at rest and during exercise in 80–100% of patients. Doppler spectra of systolic bloodflow may be used to assess stroke volume and cardiac output, by combination with the ascending aortic diameter. However, these measurements introduce a degree of inaccuracy, and as the left ventricular outflow dimensions do not change [15] during stress (except in the presence of dynamic left ventricular outflow tract obstruction), the velocity and acceleration data may be used to characterize left ventricular systolic function [16]. Accordingly, it was found that the stress-induced augmentation of aortic flow velocities of normal controls exceeded those of patients with coronary disease, particularly those with abnormal resting left ventricular function, and multivessel disease [17]. However, in a less selected group, considerable overlap was found between patients with a normal and an ischemic picture at thallium scintigraphy [18], though again the ischemic patients differed significantly from controls. These findings correspond to the limitations of examining global left ventricular functional parameters (see below), as these are relatively insensitive to small areas of ischemia, which do not compromise global cardiac function. Moreover, stress-induced alterations in global cardiac function are not specific for coronary disease. For these theoretical and practical reasons, stress Doppler examinations of systolic function have not found clinical application.

Ischemia-induced alterations of left ventricular filling may be examined by Doppler measurements of transmitral flow. The measured parameters include the peak passive (E wave) and active (A wave) filling velocities, the E:A ratio, the deceleration time of passive (E wave) flow, diastolic time intervals, and flow-velocity integrals of passive and active flow [19]. The major limitation of this approach is that stress-induced tachycardias may compromise the comparison of passive and active filling components, as the E and A waves merge at higher heart rates. This difficulty has been circumvented by the use of atrial pacing stress, which enables tachycardia to be stopped abruptly in order to interrogate left ventricular filling (see Chapter 4). Using this technique, Iliceto has demonstrated pacing-induced ischemia to correlate with diastolic dysfunction [20]. However, the relationship between stress and mitral flow is more complex than between it and aortic flow, as exercise causes an augmentation of the effective valve area rather than an increase in mitral diastolic time-velocity integral [21]. This ability of the valve orifice to change may blunt flow modifications due to ischemia and may limit the ability of diastolic flow profiles to identify coronary disease. In practical terms, the analysis of diastolic function changes has also not found wide application in clinical stress echocardiography.

Finally, color-flow Doppler may be able to contribute to the diagnosis of myocardial ischemia by documentation of stress-induced mitral regurgitation due to papillary muscle dysfunction. The practical benefit of this test has been shown for both exercise and pharmacological stress approaches [22,23]. Moreover, it may have the clinical benefit of explaining the occurrence of dyspnea disproportionate to the severity of coronary disease. The low frame-rates imposed by color-flow mapping (especially over wide sectors) are a limitation in the use of this technology during stress-induced tachycardias. This situation may constitute another area where pacing stress is of specific benefit.

2.3 Qualitative Interpretation of Stress Echocardiography

2.3.1 *General Observations on Qualitative Interpretation of Regional Function*

While some variations in the style and emphasis of performing the two-dimensional echo acquisition require a learning curve for the technician performing the test, the individual interpreting the test also has an important requirement for expertise. The length and difficulty of this process is related to the experience of the echocardiographer, but even with accomplished echocardiographers, experience varies with respect to the duration of this learning period. Picano [24] reported that a period of 6 months and 100 supervised studies was required to bring the accuracy of "novices" experienced in echocardiography (but not stress echocardiography) to the level of "experts", whose accuracy did not vary over time (Figure 2.6). However, this study was performed using dipyridamole stress echocardiography, which

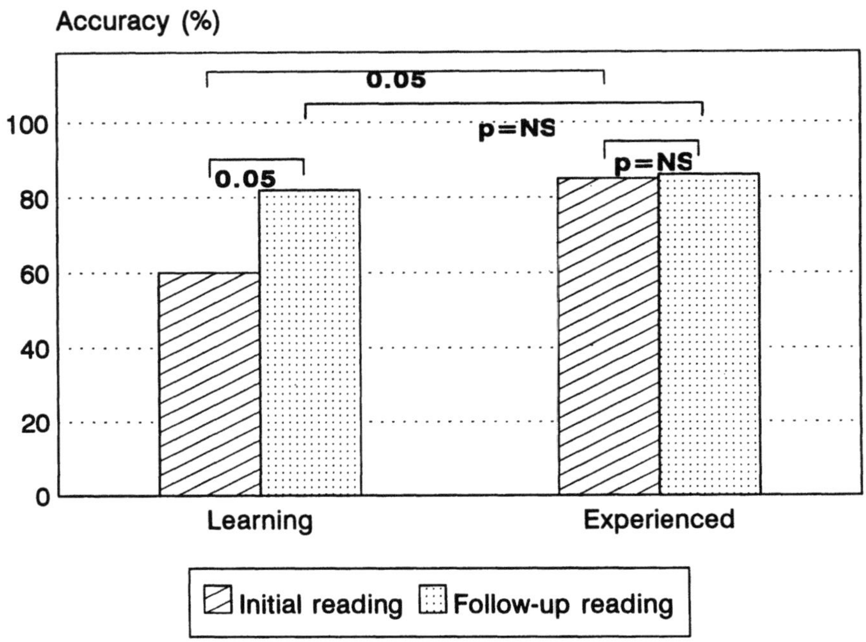

Figure 2.6. Effect of a training period on the accuracy of interpretation of stress echocardiograms by learning and experienced groups of observers (see text). Modified from Picano [24].

is a less potent inducer of ischemia than dobutamine or exercise stress – leading to less severe and more localized wall motion abnormalities, which may be more subtle to appreciate than those induced by other stresses. Moreover, the interpretations in Picano's study were obtained from video tape, and our experience suggests that it is easier to identify changes in regional function when comparing segments in a digitized, side-by-side format. Therefore, our expectation is that this learning period is somewhat shorter using exercise or dobutamine echocardiography, and image digitization. Irrespective of these details, once this expertise is achieved, stress echocardiography interpretations have proven to be highly reproducible [25].

For practical purposes, we concur with the following rules for qualitative interpretation; minor degrees of hypokinesia are not identified as ischemia (especially if only apparent at peak, and not post-exercise), abnormalities are corroborated whenever possible with another view, studies are read by multiple observers whenever possible, and reading is blinded to all other data [26]. When reviewing examinations, we rely predominantly on the digitized images, but also use video images to corroborate technically difficult studies, examine non-standard views, and to check M-mode and Doppler analyses. The first step is to check that images are triggered correctly and the pre-, peak- and post-stress views are comparable – if not, little reliance

Table 2.1. Interpretation of stress echocardiography for the diagnosis of coronary artery disease.

Diagnosis	Resting function	Peak/post-stress regional function
Normal	Normal	Hyperkinesis
Ischemic	Normal	Reduction compared with rest Reduction compared with other hyperkinetic segments Delayed contraction
	Hypokinetic	Reduction compared with rest Failure to improve (? – see text)
Infarction	Akinetic/dyskinetic	Not interpretable for ischemia (see text)

should be placed on the digitized data, and the video may be used exclusively in such situations. We then briefly review the whole study, first checking if wall motion is normal at rest, then to see if there are obvious changes in cavity size (suggesting multivessel disease) or cavity shape. Such changes occur in the presence of severe ischemia, and the most important evaluation is based upon comparison of regional function at rest and stress. In order to standardize these findings, the left ventricle is usually divided into a number of segments, defined by various landmarks. The American Society of Echocardiography recommendations have been modified (Figure 2.7) to comprise 16 segments (septal, lateral, anterior and inferior at the apex, with these segments as well as anteroseptal, and posterior segments at the base and mid-papillary muscle level). Function at rest and stress is compared in each segment both by examining the continuous cine-loop and then frame-by-frame, using the digital images and paying particular attention to contraction during the first part of systole (especially if there is excessive rotational or translational movement). The following are offered as a guideline to facilitate decision-making about what constitutes normal, ischemic and infarcted myocardium (Table 2.1).

2.3.2 *Interpretation of Resting Function*

Regional wall motion at rest may be classified as dyskinetic, akinetic, hypokinetic or normal. The presence of abnormal regional function at rest implies previous infarction, but unfortunately, hypokinesia may be seen as a normal variant [27]. Hypokinetic segments, therefore, should not be identified as being infarcted, on the basis that residual contraction implies th

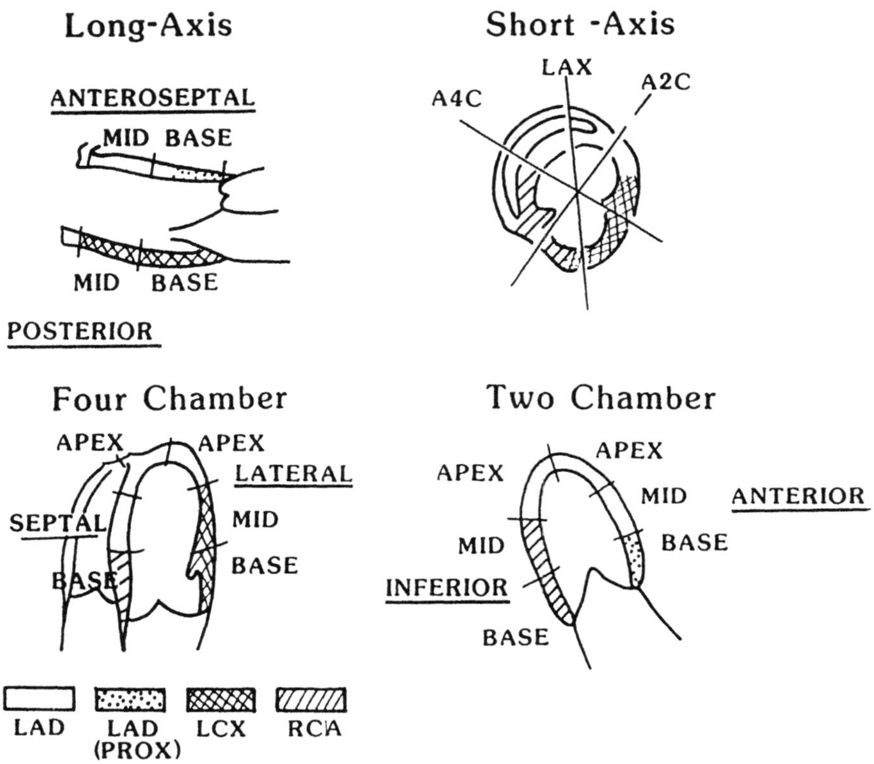

Figure 2.7. Segmentation of the left ventricle, showing assumed perfusion territories of the 3 major coronary vessels in parasternal long axis, short-axis, apical four-chamber and apical two-chamber views.

Other difficulties arise with this algorithm for the echocardiographic diagnosis of infarction. First, small (especially non Q-wave) infarcts may not cause any wall motion abnormality, or cause hypokinesia, which is not recognised as infarction. Second, problems may occur in the distinction of severe hypokinesia (non-infarcted) from akinesia (infarcted). A useful guide is to identify akinesia based upon endocardial excursion < 2 mm, and hypokinesia with endocardial excursion < 5 mm, although this simplifies the problems inherent in attempts to quantitate regional movement (see below). For example, regions which fail to thicken or which move only in late systole (after movement of the adjacent myocardium), may be moving passively, and should be considered as akinetic irrespective of endocardial excursion. Third, even the presence of akinesis or dyskinesis may not correlate with infarction in a pathologic sense, and such regions may actually consist of viable tissue. Thus, if the clinical question pertains to myocardial viability, a different algorithm should be used for qualitative interpretation. In these circumstances, the diagnosis may be tempered by the thickness of the involved

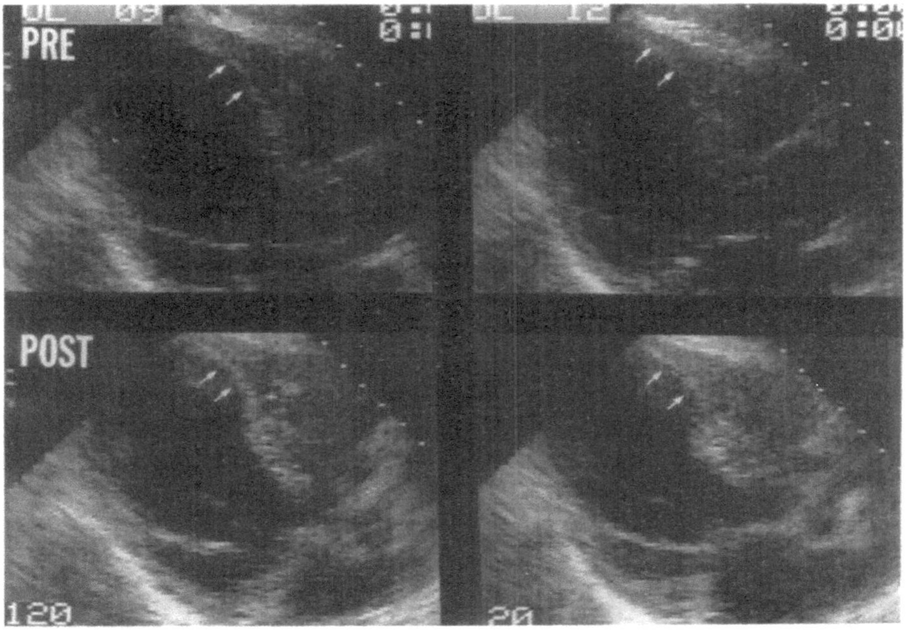

Figure 2.8. Pre- and post-exercise images in diastole (left) and systole (right) showing infarction of the anteroseptal wall. Note that in addition to akinesis and failure to respond to stress, the region (arrowed) is thinned and echodense. Reproduced with permission of the American Journal of Cardiac Imaging.

myocardium – thinned and echodense tissue corroborates the diagnosis of infarction (Figure 2.8), though myocardium of normal thickness does not

sequel of myocardial ischemia, which is readily and reproducibly identified if akinesia or dyskinesia are induced. Stress-induced hypokinesia is more difficult to identify, and use of a reference marker on the screen may assist in its detection, particularly if it is relative to hyperkinesia in other segments (as opposed to an absolute deterioration compared with rest). Moreover, using quantitative techniques [29], considerable variability has been identified in regional wall motion at peak exercise, and regional hypokinesis may occur in normal individuals. In the light of these considerations, the detection of more subtle indices (tardokinesis and reduced thickening) together with hypokinesis may confirm the diagnosis of ischemia. Unfortunately, an appreciation of myocardial thickening requires good quality images with definition of the epicardium; it is often only readily apparent in the septum. The perception of tardokinesis is facilitated by the improved stop-frame images permitted by image digitization, but nonetheless remains relative and somewhat subjective. To avoid false positives due to inhomogeneous updating of the video image, we have arbitrarily selected a delay of 100 msec (2 stop frames) as the minimum to justify a diagnosis of ischemia on these grounds.

The diagnosis of ischemia in segments with abnormal resting function is more difficult to interpret, and may to some extent depend upon the stress agent. Using bicycle or dobutamine echocardiography, if a segment is identified as infarcted by akinesia or dyskinesia at rest, we do not classify a further deterioration of function as ischemia [30], as increased loading may be responsible for such a response. This may not be true of vasodilator stress echocardiography, where ischemia is characterized as a new or worsening wall motion abnormality [31]. The diagnosis of ischemia in segments showing resting hypokinesis is probably the most difficult and controversial interpretation. Myocardium with resting hypokinesis but showing a stress-induced improvement is identified as normal. From a theoretical standpoint, a further deterioration is consistent with ischemia, though in practical terms, this may be hard to identify confidently. The use of a side-by-side cine loop analysis greatly facilitates this interpretation, and use of a reference marker on the screen is invaluable in comparing minor changes in the severity of hypokinesis. Finally, there is no consensus regarding the diagnosis in hypokinetic regions which fail to improve function – we have previously characterized these as ischemic, based upon the absence of hyperkinesis, but this definition (and its opposite) are unsupported experimentally.

2.3.4 *Factors other than Coronary Disease Influencing Regional Function*

Non-coronary factors may influence regional cardiac function. The hemodynamic status of the patient may impact upon the recognition of wall motion abnormalities; pressure loads (for example, hypertension) increase local wall stress and enhance the recognition of dysfunctional regions, while reduction of afterload (for example, by mitral regurgitation) may reduce wall stress and make regional dysfunction less prominent.

Local factors potentially causing false positive scans for ischemia include abnormal electrical activation (pacing, left bundle branch block, Wolf-Parkinson-White syndrome), abnormal septal movement due to previous cardiac surgery or right ventricular volume overload, and heterogeneities related to cardiomyopathies, aortic and mitral regurgitation. Areas adjacent to zones of myocardial infarction may be tethered by the akinetic infarcted zone and consequently fail to improve function with stress, or even appear dyskinetic if the infarct bulges during stress. In this circumstance, it is difficult to distinguish peri-infarct ischemia and tethering, though this distinction may be clarified by careful examination of wall thickening. A similar process may account for apparent wall motion abnormalities in the basal inferior wall, close to the plane of the mitral valve, where isolated wall motion abnormalities require cautious interpretation. Other causes of false positive and false negative studies are addressed further in Chapter 3.

2.3.5 *The Stress Echocardiogram Report*

In addition to the detection of ischemia-induced wall motion disturbances, stress echocardiography may give prognostically-important information regarding the degree of coronary disease. This may be inferred from the site, extent (number of abnormal segments), severity (segmental wall motion score), time of onset and offset of ischemia, and the effect of ischemia on global left ventricular function. The report should reflect these other findings in addition to identifying the presence or absence of coronary disease. We report stress echocardiograms as follows;

i. Resting images

- resting wall motion
- structural abnormalities which may account for the patient's symptoms

ii. Stress images

- presence, site, extent, and severity of abnormal function
- time of onset and duration after stress

iii. Segmental function

- wall motion score at rest, and during or after stress

iv. Global analysis

- function at rest and stress, based on qualitative evaluation, wall motion scoring, or ejection fraction calculations.

2.4 Quantitative Analysis of Regional Function

There are global and regional quantitative approaches to the evaluation of left ventricular wall motion. These may be further divided into semi- and fully-quantitative categories.

A semi-quantitative regional approach is widely used for the reporting of exercise echocardiograms, and is an extension of the qualitative method described above. Instead of identifying improvement or deterioration within regions, application of this method is based upon scoring regional function. Various scoring systems have been used; we use a modification of the American Society of Echocardiography segmentation described by Broderick [32]. With this, a score of 1 is given for normal regions, with scores of 2, 3 and 4 for hypokinesis, akinesis and dyskinesis, 5 for aneursym, and 6 and 7 for akinesis or dyskinesis with thinning, respectively. By averaging the scores of individual segments, a "score index" may be obtained, which gives a semi-quantitative index of global systolic function, analogous to the ejection fraction, with similar prognostic significance [33].

While these scoring methods go some way towards countering the criticism of subjectivity, they do not truly measure function independent of the observer. Global systolic function may be quantitated by tracing systolic and diastolic contours for the calculation of ventricular volumes and ejection fraction [34]. Unfortunately, however, ejection fraction is an imperfect measure of contractility, being dependent on loading conditions and heart-rate. An alternative and less loading-dependent measure is the peak systolic pressure-end systolic volume ratio [35]. Nonetheless, all global indices share the problem of being relatively insensitive to mild ischemia, as well as being non-specific for coronary disease.

The quantitation of regional function involves tracing of endocardial (and for some methods, epicardial) interfaces, their superimposition using a fixed or floating reference system, and measurement of the selected parameters. There are potential problems at each step. Tracing of contours is dependent upon border definition of good quality – in our experience of bicycle and post-treadmill stress, only 40 to 50% of images have adequate image quality for tracing of the endocardial contours in systole and diastole – an experience which contrasts with the ability to subjectively interpret over 90 to 95% of studies in cine-loop format. Moreover, the usual reliance on apical views to examine most of the myocardium is limited by suboptimal edge detection caused by the parallel orientation of the echocardiographic beam with the endocardium, a problem which may be circumvented by use of the subcostal window during erect bicycle stress [35], but at the cost of limiting the amount of myocardium examined. Moreover, even with this time-consuming activity, the technique is not objective, as some subjectivity is inherent in tracing the borders. The second major problem relates to choices as to whether or not a fixed or floating frame of reference should be used in order to compensate for rotational or translational movement of the heart [36]. Failure to correct

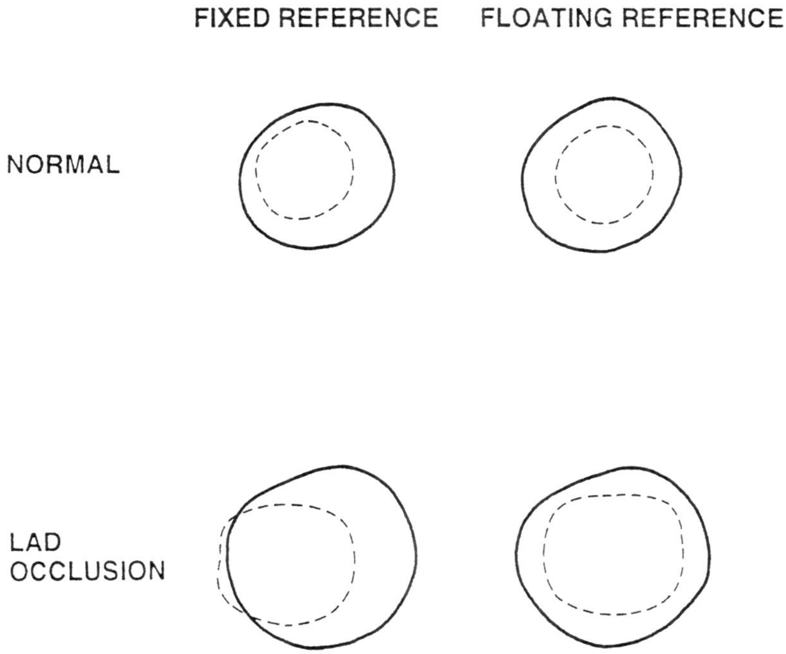

Figure 2.9. Benefits and disadvantages of fixed and floating reference systems, as applied to short axis views. A fixed system does not compensate for translational and rotational cardiac movement, so that superimposition of systolic (dashed line) and diastolic images may suggest abnormal function even in normal ventricles (upper left). Superimposition of images based upon the center of mass (upper right) corrects for this extrinsic cardiac movement. However, the same process may inappropriately correct ischemia-induced wall motion abnormalities (lower right).

for such movements may cause false positives, but their correction may hinder the detection of milder abnormalities (Figure 2.9). Finally, as systole is temporally heterogeneous among different myocardial regions, not just one but several frames should be traced to form a composite picture of maximum systole – a tedious and time-consuming process which is unattractive for clinical practice.

Regional function may be quantitated as thickening or endocardial excursion. While the former is more independent of cardiac translation or rotation (and hence the center of reference is of less concern), the results are difficult to correlate with those of other modalities, and most importantly, the feasibility of this method is limited by difficulty in tracing the epicardial border. Endocardial excursion may be measured by segmental area shrinkage, perimeter shrinkage, or radial change. A modification of the latter, involving the center-line method [37] has become the most widely accepted approach.

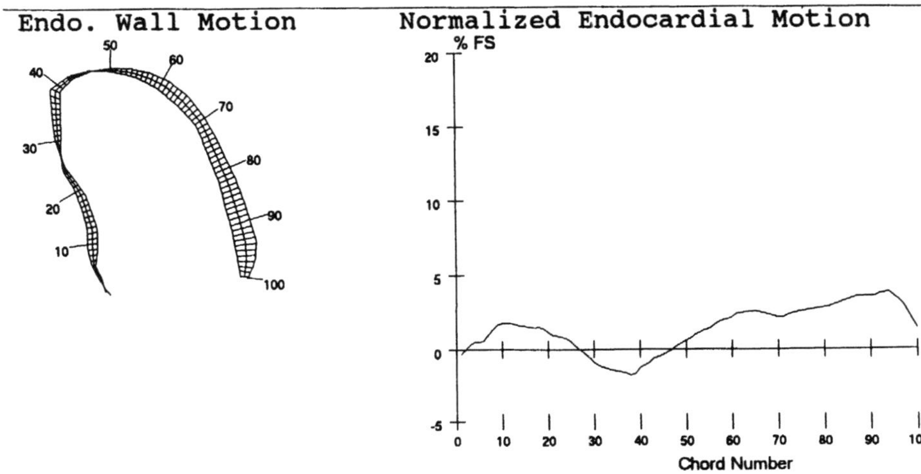

Figure 2.10. Centerline method for quantitation of regional left ventricular dysfunction. A line is centered between diastolic and systolic outlines, and the excursion around this line is measured in 100 chords, placed perpendicular to the endocardium. The results may be graphed to portray excursion on a segmental basis; in this example, the apical septum demonstrates dyskinesis, which is evidenced as a negative deflection from chords 26–47.

This method first requires tracing and superimposition of systolic and diastolic images. A center-line is drawn midway between these profiles, and chords are arranged perpendicular to the centerline. Chord lengths, normalized for body size and the diastolic perimeter length, are then expressed as a function of location (on the x-axis), and compared with a normal range (Figure 2.10). Although favorable results have been obtained using this fully quantitative approach for the interpretation of regional function [35], it is time-consuming and at present, not clearly superior to the qualitative methods. At present, therefore, the quantitative approach remains a research rather than a clinical tool at most centers.

2.5 New Approaches to the Interpretation of Stress Echocardiography

As described above, stress echocardiography is currently highly dependent upon subjective analysis, and quantitation presents a multiplicity of problems. Nonetheless, there is an appreciation that the full potential of this technique will only be realized as a routine test when the results are quantitated, preferably with a degree of automation. The first steps must concern image enhancement and edge detection, and there have recently been some encouraging advances. Problems arising from translational movement may now be corrected by superimposition of colorized diastolic and systolic images, without algorithms based upon the center of mass [38]. Color Doppler imaging has been applied to the definition of acceleration of the myocardial walls [39], with improvement of image quality. These advances may facilitate the quantitation of regional function.

Significant developments in 2–dimensional echocardiography are occurring in the sphere of backscatter analysis and tissue characterization. Both the mean amplitude of ultrasonic backscatter [40], and its cyclic variation during systole and diastole [41] have been altered by ischemia in animal models. The application of this technology to the clinical arena is undergoing preliminary development. Picano [42] has recently reported that videodensitometry may be used to show that asynergic myocardium due to ischemia demonstrates increased echodensity, although changes in cyclic variation could only be obtained during coronary angioplasty. Clearly, this system will need to corroborate the presence of ischemia in segments which are hypokinetic: greater sensitivity is likely to be obtained when reflected signal intensity can be directly analysed without video processing. In the future, an appreciation of echodensity and backscatter variation may then assist in the qualitative interpretation of wall excursion, timing, and thickening.

The difference between the backscatter characteristics of myocardium and blood has recently been used to obtain automatic detection and tracking of the left ventricular cavity [43]. On-line quantitation of left ventricular volumes has been utilized during dobutamine echocardiography [44], and groups with "normal" and "abnormal" responses may be thus defined, although no correlates with coronary anatomy or regional left ventricular function have been reported. However, our initial impression is that automated edge detection does not yet enhance the accuracy of regional analysis for stress echocardiography.

Finally, the development of transpulmonary contrast agents may further enhance the ability to localize the endocardial border. In addition, contrast echocardiography may permit quantitation of myocardial perfusion. Echocardiography may eventually offer a means of evaluating both perfusion and function using the same technique, at both rest and stress.

2.6 Pitfalls in the Performance and Interpretation of Stress Echocardiography

The above sections have been directed towards practical issues regarding the performance and interpretation of stress echocardiograms. The novice practitioner also needs to prepare for potential sources of inaccuracy, which may pertain to the physician supervising the test, patient, echocardiogram, digitizer or image interpretation.

It is critical that the appropriate form of stress is chosen to answer a particular clinical question. For example, the functional evaluation of the heart after myocardial infarction involves issues pertaining to myocardial viability, suggesting that a dobutamine test may be the optimal choice. In contrast, in a patient without previous infarction, who is able to exercise maximally, exercise echocardiography may be the optimal choice. Issues regarding optimization of tests for individual patients are still being investigated, and are discussed in later chapters.

With respect to patient factors, the limitations posed by poorly echogenic patients are real, although probably overstated. Of greater importance are patient-related factors which limit the ability to induce ischemia, including inability to exercise maximally or tolerate maximal doses of dobutamine (see Chapters 3 and 4) and ingestion of anti-anginal drugs. The importance of the latter is determined by the reason for the test; investigation on therapy is appropriate if the clinical question pertains to the efficacy of treatment for the control of angina, but it is inappropriate if the test is performed for diagnostic purposes. The effect of anti-anginal therapy on the development of dipyridamole-induced wall motion abnormalities has been studied by Lattanzi [45]. Using a placebo-controlled design, this study demonstrated that betablockers and calcium antagonists reduced the sensitivity of dipyridamole echocardiography from 92% to 67% and 85% to 62%, respectively. In 3 patients treated with both agents, the sensitivity was reduced from 100% (on placebo) to 33% (on treatment).

Echocardiographic factors leading to erroneous results are avoidable. Apart from technically difficult studies, they include the use of inadequate equipment or insufficiently trained technicians. Ischemia may be missed in these situations by failure to visualize the abnormal segment, or delayed imaging after ischemia has resolved. Similarly, the digitizer may be responsible for problems if ECG gating is not optimized, or if used inexpertly. The greatest potential pitfalls, however, relate to the interpretation of studies. Failure to appreciate the subtle manifestations of ischemia (tardokinesis and hypokinesis), as well as over-interpretation of basal wall motion abnormalities are avoidable with adequate training. However, some interpretations are difficult even for experts – these include studies involving abnormal septal movement of non-ischemic origin (due to coronary graft surgery or left bundle branch block), the distinction of peri-infarct ischemia from tethering of adjacent myocardium to the infarct zone, and interpretation of suboptimal images. Images involving extensive translational movement require particularly careful attention, with examination of the first half of the cardiac cycle and careful corroboration of findings between views.

2.7 Conclusion

The development of stress echocardiography has paralleled improvements on echocardiographic technology and image processing. Even the best equipment, however, cannot substitute for expertise in both image acquisition and interpretation. The achievement of results comparable to those in the literature is therefore dependent upon the training of the echocardiographer.

References

1. Presti CF, Armstrong WF, Feigenbaum H. Comparison of echocardiography at peak exercise and after bicycle exercise in evaluation of patients with known or suspected coronary artery disease. J Am Soc Echo 1988;1:119–26.
2. Ginzton LE. Stress·echocardiography and myocardial contrast echocardiography. Cardiol Clin 1989;7:493–509.
3. Feigenbaum H. The echocardiographic examination. In: Feigenbaum H, editor. Echocardiography. 4th ed. Philadelphia: Lea & Febinger, 1986.
4. Skorton DJ, Collins SM, Kerber RE. Digital image processing and analysis in echocardiography. In: Collins SM, Skorton DJ. Cardiac imaging and image processing. New York: McGraw-Hill, 1986.
5. Feigenbaum H. Exercise echocardiography. J Am Soc Echo 1988;1:161–6.
6. Marwick T, D'Hondt A-M, Mairesse G *et al.* Should patients able to exercise undergo exercise or dobutamine echocardiography? [abstract] Eur Heart J 1993;14:454.
7. Sevilla DC, Dohrmann ML, Somelofski CA, Wawrzynski RP, Wagner NB, Wagner GS. Invalidation of the resting electrocardiogram obtained via exercise electrode sites as a standard 12–lead recording. Am J Cardiol 1989;63:35–9.
8. Heng MK, Simard M, Lake R, Udhoji VH. Exercise two-dimensional echocardiography for diagnosis of coronary artery disease. Am J Cardiol 1984;54:502–7.
9. Mitamura H, Ogawa S, Hori S *et al.* Two-dimensional echocardiographic analysis of wall motion abnormalities during handgrip exercise in patients with coronary artery disease. Am J Cardiol 1981;48:711–7.
10. Mancini GBJ, Peterson KL, Gregoratos G, Higgins CB. Effects of atrial pacing on global and regional left ventricular function in coronary heart disease assessed by digital intravenous ventriculography. Am J Cardiol 1984;53:456–61.
11. Iliceto S, Sorino M, D'Ambrosio G *et al.* Detection of coronary artery disease by two-dimensional echocardiography and transesophageal atrial pacing. J Am Coll Cardiol 1985;5:1188–97.
12. Lambertz H, Kreis A, Trumper H, Hanrath P. Simultaneous transesophageal atrial pacing and transesophageal echocardiography: A new method of stress echocardiography. J Am Coll Cardiol 1990;16:1143–53.
13. Ginzton LE, Conant R, Brizendine M, Lee F, Mena I, Laks M. Exercise subcostal two-dimensional echocardiography: A new method of segmental wall motion abnormality. Am J Cardiol 1984;53:805–11.
14. Fisher EA, Stahl JA, Budd JH, Goldman ME. Transesophageal echocardiography: procedures and clinical application. J Am Coll Cardiol 1991;18:1333–48.
15. Ihlen H, Amlie JP, Dale J *et al.* Determination of cardiac output by Doppler echocardiography. Br Heart J 1984;51:54–60.
16. Sabbah, HN, Khaja F, Brymer JF *et al.* Non-invasive evaluation of left ventricular performance based on peak aortic blood flow acceleration measured by a continuous-wave Doppler velocity meter. Circulation 1986;74:323–9.
17. Bryg RJ, Labovitz AJ, Mehdirad AA *et al.* Effect of coronary artery disease on Doppler-derived parameters of aortic flow during upright exercise. Am J Cardiol 1986;58:14–9.
18. Harrison MR, Smith MD, Friedman BJ, De Maria AN. Uses and limitaions of exercise Doppler echocardiography in the diagnosis of ischemic heart disease. J Am Coll Cardiol 1987;10:809–15.
19. Nishimura RA, Abel MD, Hatle LK, Tajik AJ. Assessment of diastolic function of the heart: Background and current applications of Doppler echocardiography. Part II Clinical studies. Mayo Clin Proc 1989;64:181–204.
20. Iliceto S, Amico A, Marangelli V, D'Ambrosio G, Rizzon P. Doppler echocardiographic evaluation of the effect of atrial pacing-induced ischemia on left ventricular filling in patients with coronary artery disease. J Am Coll Cardiol 1988;11:953–61.

21. Rassi A, Crawford MH, Richards KL, Miller JF. Differing mechanisms of exercise flow augmentation at the mitral and aortic valves. Circulation 1988;77:543–51.
22. Zachariah ZP, Hsuing MC, Nanda NC, Kan MN, Gatewood Jr RP. Color Doppler assessment of mitral regurgitation induced by supine exercise in ischemic heart disease. Am J Cardiol 1987;59:1266–70.
23. Mazeika P, Nihoyannopoulos P, Joshi J, Oakley CM. Evaluation of dipyridamole-Doppler echocardiography for detection of myocardial ischemia and coronary artery disease. Am J Cardiol 1991;68:478–84.
24. Picano E, Lattanzi F, Orlandini A, Marini C, L'Abbate A. Stress echocardiography and the human factor: The importance of being expert. J Am Coll Cardiol 1991;17:666–9.
25. Oberman A, Fan PH, Nanda NC *et al.* Reproducibility of two-dimensional exercise echocardiography. J Am Coll Cardiol 1989;14:923–8.
26. Picano E, Lattanzi F. Dipyridamole echocardiography: A new diagnostic window on coronary artery disease. Circulation 1991;83(SupplIII):19–26.
27. Pandian NG, Skorton DJ, Collins SM, Falsetti HL, Burke ER, Kerber RE. Heterogeneity of left ventricular segmental wall thickening and excursion in 2–dimensional echocardiograms of normal human subjects. Am J Cardiol 1983;51:1667–73.
28. Pierard LA, De Landsheere C, Berthe C, Rigo P, Kulbertus HE. Identification of viable myocardium by echocardiography during dobutamine infusion in patients with myocardial infarction after thrombolytic therapy: Comparison with positron emission tomography. J Am Coll Cardiol 1990;15:1021–31.
29. Ginzton LE, Conant R, Brizendine M, Thigpen T, Laks MM. Quantitative analysis of segmental wall motion during maximal upright dynamic exercise: variability in normal adults. Circulation 1986;73:268–75.
30. Marwick T, Salcedo EE, Stewart WJ. Exercise echocardiographic and Doppler evaluation of left ventricular function. Am J Card Imaging 1991;5:281–90.
31. Picano E, Lattanzi F, Massini M, Distante A, L'Abbate A. High dose dipyridamole echocardiography test in effort angina pectoris. J Am Coll Cardiol 1986;8:848–54.
32. Broderick T, Sawada S, Armstrong WF *et al.* Improvement in rest and exercise-induced wall motion abnormalities after coronary angioplasty: An exercise echocardiographic study. J Am Coll Cardiol 1990;15:591–9.
33. Nishimura RA, Reeder GS, Miller FA *et al.* Prognostic value of predischarge 2–dimensional echocardiogram after acute myocardial infarction. Am J Cardiol 1984;53:429–32.
34. Stamm RB, Carabello BA, Moyers DL, Martin RP. Two-dimensional echocardiographic measurement of left ventricular ejection fraction: Prospective analysis of what constitutes an adequate determination. Am Heart J 1982;104:136–44.
35. Ginzton LE, Laks M, Brizendine M *et al.* Non-invasive measurement of the rest and exercise peak systolic pressure/end-systolic volume ratio: a sensitive two-dimensional echocardiographic indicator of left ventricular function. J Am Coll Cardiol 1984;4:509–16.
36. Force TL, Folland ED, Aebischer N, Sharma S, Parisi AF. Echocardiographic assessment of ventricular function. In: Marcus ML, Schelbert HR, Skorton DJ, Wolf GL, editors. Cardiac imaging. Philadelphia: WB Saunders, 1991.
37. Sheehan FH, Stewart AK, Dodge HT *et al.* Variability in the measurement of regional left ventricular wall motion from contrast angiograms. Circulation 1983;68;550–9.
38. Bates JR, Segar DS, Ryan T, Sawada SG, Fitch GN, Feigenbaum H. Colorized wall motion analysis to detect and correct for translation during upright bicycle stress echocardiography [abstract]. J Am Coll Cardiol 1993;21:275A.
39. Guell-Peris FJ, Groundstroem KW, Sutherland GR *et al.* Myocardial imaging by colour Doppler coded velocity mapping – A new method for the assessment of myocardial contractility [abstract]. J Am Coll Cardiol 1993;21:276A.
40. Schnittger I, Vieli A, Heiserman JE *et al.* Ultrasonic tissue characerization: detection of acute myocardial ischemia in dogs. Circulation 1985;72:193–9.
41. Glueck RM, Motley JG, Miller JG, Sobel BE. Effects of coronary artery occlusion and

reperfusion on cardiac cycle-dependent variation of myocardial ultrasonic backscatter. Circ Res 1985;56:683–9.

42. Picano E, Faletra F, Marini C *et al.* Increased echodensity of transiently asynergic myocardium in humans: a novel echocardiographic sign of myocardial ischemia. J Am Coll Cardiol 1993;21:199–207.
43. Perez JE, Waggoner AD, Barzilai B, Melton HE, Miller JG, Sobel BE. On-line assessment of ventricular function by automatic boundary detection and ultrasonic backscatter imaging. J Am Coll Cardiol 1992;19:313–20.
44. Perez JE, Waggoner AD, Davila-Roman VG, Cardona H, Miller JG. On-line quantification of ventricular function during dobutamine stress echocardiography. Eur Heart J 1992;13:1669–76.
45. Lattanzi F, Picano E, Bolognese L *et al.* Inhibition of dipyridamole-induced ischemia by antianginal therapy in humans: Correlation with exercise echocardiography. Circulation 1991;83:1256–62.

3. Exercise Echocardiography

The combination of exercise with two-dimensional echocardiography was the first reported form of stress echocardiography. It remains, arguably, the optimal combination of stress with echocardiography. This chapter will examine methodological aspects and the accuracy of this test in the detection of coronary disease. Comparisons with the stress ECG and other stress-imaging combinations will be addressed in subsequent chapters.

3.1 Methodologies of Exercise Echocardiography

The equipment required for performance of exercise echocardiography is a high quality echocardiography machine, preferably with on-line connection to a digitizer, in addition to standard stress equipment (treadmill, upright or supine bicycle). The study requires the presence of two technicians, one to perform the exercise test and monitor the hemodynamic and ECG response to exercise, and the other to acquire the echocardiographic images. The technique of performing the test differs according to the exercise methodology selected.

3.1.1 *Treadmill Exercise Stress*

Treadmill stress echocardiography [1] is based upon the comparison of pre- and post-exercise data (usually the parasternal long- and short-axis and apical four- and two-chamber views). We normally perform diagnostic exercise echocardiograms after abstention from anti-anginal therapy for at least one day, as these drugs may prevent the development of myocardial ischemia. The patient is prepared for exercise in the usual fashion. Resting images are obtained in the standard left lateral position, digitized on-line and saved in a quad-screen format before exercise begins. ECG electrodes (usually leads V2 and V5 only) may need to be relocated prior to stress if they interfere with the echocardiographic windows [2]. An appropriate stress protocol is selected, based upon the clinical status of the patient, who then proceeds to exercise in the standard fashion, the test being modified only to obtain images as rapidly as possible. Hence, no "cool-down" period is interposed between peak exercise and lying down, as any delay in post-exercise imaging may be

T.H. Marwick, Stress Echocardiography, 39–59.

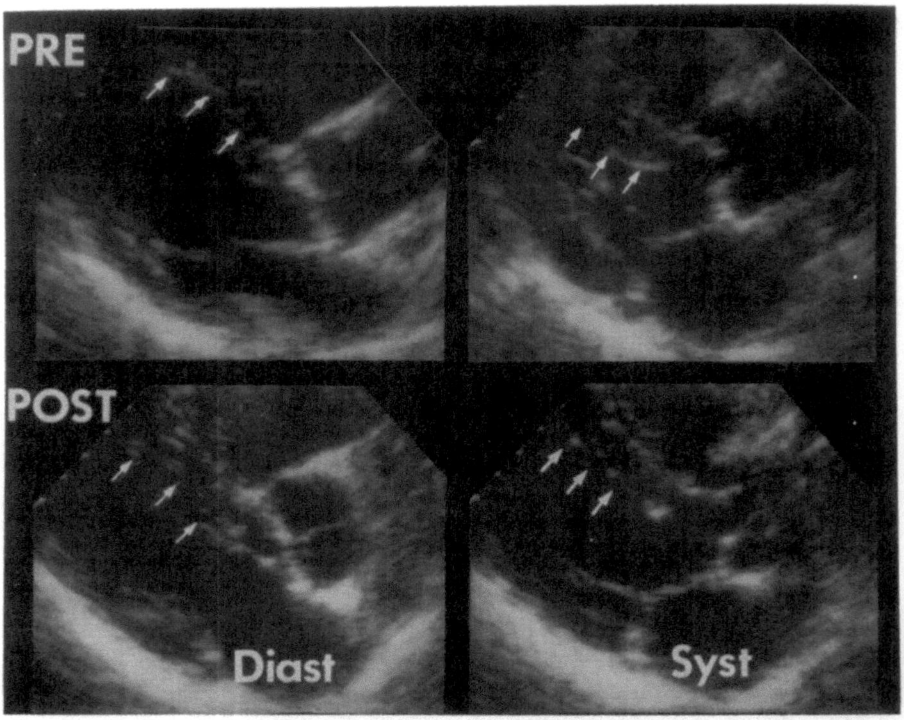

Figure 3.1. Pre- and post-treadmill exercise systolic and diastolic images demonstrating normal resting function, with anteroseptal ischemia (arrows) after stress. Reproduced with permission of the Journal of the American College of Cardiology.

matched by a loss of sensitivity, particularly for the diagnosis of milder or well-collateralized coronary disease [3]. The process of getting off the treadmill should take no more than 20 seconds with practice, enabling rapid resumption of imaging in the left lateral position as soon as possible after peak exercise. As discussed in Chapter 2, post-stress imaging is greatly facilitated by on-line image digitization, as the formation of sequential cine-loops allows the technician to be confident that at least one cardiac cycle of good quality has been obtained. The use of a digitizer also enables selection of an optimal end-expiratory image from sequential cine-loops after exercise. Finally, selected pre- and post-exercise cine loops are re-mixed digitally [2], conventionally with resting images displayed to the left of the post-exercise images (Figure 3.1).

3.1.2 *Bicycle Exercise Stress*

Bicycle stress is usually performed in the upright position [4], although supine bicycle stress has recently been combined with echocardiography [5]. As with treadmill stress, the patient undergoes routine preparation for exercise. Resting supine images are acquired and digitized as described above. The protocol then deviates from usual echocardiographic practice, with acquisition of images in the upright position on the bicycle. This usually permits apical images of high quality, which may be supplemented by subcostal views [4]. Satisfactory parasternal views may be obtained at rest if the patient is instructed to lean forwards and exhale, and these images often improve during stress. The acquisition of resting upright views has two benefits; first (and paradoxically), they may offer better image quality, and second, they offer a resting image with the same orientation as views acquired during exercise, thus permitting comparisons of wall motion in peak and post-stress views in as close as possible to equivalent regions. Exercise is commenced, and the standard views may be obtained at each stage of exercise, digitized and recorded on video tape. Although older digital acquisition systems only permitted the archiving of peak exercise images, the availability of larger amounts of computer memory has permitted saving digital data at each level of exercise. Despite the attractions of peak imaging, post-stress images should also be obtained, as some wall motion abnormalities may only be recognized in these supine images, due either to technical problems with peak data acquisition (suboptimal upright image quality and conclusion of exercise after having saved peak data), or the provocation of abnormal function by increasing preload on lying down post-stress. Finally, after exercise, the best pre-peak, peak- and post-exercise line loops are selected and mixed with the appropriate (supine or upright) resting images.

3.1.3 *Selection of the Optimal Exercise Stress*

The exercise methodology of choice for stress echocardiography remains undefined, and treadmill and bicycle exercise echocardiography each have their advocates. Pre- and post-treadmill protocols are probably the most widely used. Their main advantage is that image acquisition is technically less demanding than during bicycle stress, as the circumstances most closely resemble those of routine echocardiography; the patient is supine and relatively immobile. The disadvantage of this approach is that, although efforts have been made to image the heart during treadmill stress [6], in the hands of most practitioners, the examination is limited to "snapshots" of the heart before and after exercise. The delay between peak exercise and the completion of post-exercise imaging is probably of limited importance (see below).

Bicycle protocols involving imaging at peak exercise are effective not only for diagnosing the presence or absence of ischemia at peak stress, but also for identifying the time of onset of ischemia, which may be a useful index of the physiologic severity of coronary disease. Moreover, several imaging considerations favor use of the cycle ergometer for stress echocardiography. First, the use of peak rather than post-exercise imaging may avoid false negative studies due to rapid resolution of ischemia. Second, images acquired in the upright position are often of surprisingly good quality, and in individuals with suboptimal supine echocardiographic windows the availability of additional upright views may materially enhance the interpretation of the study. Indeed, the decision about the presence or absence of coronary disease is made on the basis of double the amount of data (peak- and post-exercise) than are available using treadmill exercise. Third, the capacity to define the time of onset of abnormal wall motion, and follow its progression over time may deliver more pathophysiologic data about the severity of disease than is available from the pre- and post-exercise "snapshot" available with treadmill protocols. These benefits are bought at the cost of technical difficulty and some compromise in specificity (see below). In addition to these technical problems, maximal exertion on a cycle ergometer may be limited by fatigue or leg discomfort without achieving peak heart rate or maximal aerobic capacity [7], especially in countries such as the USA and Britain, where bicycles are not widely used in everyday life. Thus, although some patients – for example those with claudication or balance disturbances – may exercise better on a bicycle, treadmill exertion is believed to more reliably stress all subjects, producing similar oxygen requirements per kilogram at comparable workloads, irrespective of fitness considerations. This perceived benefit of treadmill exercise is notwithstanding the fact that, at an equivalent workload, bicycle exercise may be associated with higher blood pressure and rate-pressure product than treadmill stress [8].

Supine bicycle stress permits the entire protocol to be performed in the left lateral position – which is the ideal situation for imaging. However, this form of stress does not reflect normal physiology, and the issue of feasibility may also pertain to the performance of supine bicycle stress, as patients often experience difficulty in performing maximal exercise in this position. Supine bicycle stress offers a potential for increased oxygen consumption (due to greater maximum blood pressure and rate-pressure product, together with the increased venous return), reflected by enhancement of anginal and ST segment responses in the supine position [9]. However, these benefits of supine exercise may never be realized if the subject becomes fatigued prematurely.

The selection of one or other of these alternatives is essentially a trade-off between image quality and feasibility (which are greater with supine imaging), and the resolution of ischemia following maximal stress (which may influence results if peak imaging cannot be performed). The time-course of ischemia reflects its duration and severity. Patients with multivessel coronary disease have been documented to demonstrate continuing abnormal wall motion for up to 30 minutes after exercise, while patients with milder disease [10] or extensive collateralization [11] do not show persisting wall motion abnormalities. Not surprisingly, during bicycle stress echocardiography [3] and nuclear ventriculography [11], regional dysfunction is more frequently observed at peak stress than after stress (Figure 3.2), suggesting that protocols offering peak stress images should be more sensitive than those (like treadmill exercise) involving post-stress imaging only. However, this would only confer a clear benefit for bicycle over treadmill exercise if the two stresses were analogous with respect to their ischemic potential, which may not be so, as exercise is limited by fatigue more frequently with the bicycle. Moreover, the ischemic period may be shorter after bicycle exercise, causing the phenomenon of lower sensitivity with post-exercise imaging to be more prominent in this situation. Indeed, the only direct comparison between bicycle and treadmill stress echocardiography reported to date suggests that there is only a minor difference in sensitivity between peak bicycle and post-treadmill methodologies for inducing ischemia [12]. This gain may be at the cost of lower specificity, probably due to artifactual interpretation of wall motion abnormalities, due to movements of the heart and body. Post-bicycle imaging avoids this problem, but at the cost of lower sensitivity.

In conclusion, while each form of stress has its particular advantages, their overall accuracies are similar, with perhaps minor benefits in terms of sensitivity for the bicycle and specificity for the treadmill (see below), although a direct comparison in a large number of patients would be necessary to confirm this. To a large extent, the selection of one or other stress is at present a matter of local preference and expertise.

3.2 Accuracy of Stress Echocardiography

The adequate assessment of any test for the diagnosis of coronary disease should be based upon guidelines ensuring that studies reflect clinical practice [13]. The most important considerations are that the study group should be as representative and as unselected as possible. Use of a representative group precludes selection of studies on the basis of image quality. It also prevents studying the extremes of the spectrum of patients with severe coronary disease in the sensitivity group, and comparison with normal controls in the specificity group. Study designs comparing the findings of stress echocardiography with coronary anatomy are necessarily biased towards a group with severe enough coronary disease to warrant angiography. However, care must be made to avoid an additional (post-test) referral bias. This process is characterized by a pattern of high test sensitivity (only patients with positive test results proceed to angiography) and low specificity (the few normal angiograms in the series being requested because of false positive test results).

The results of comparisons between exercise echocardiography and angiography [5,10,14–35] are reviewed in Table 3.1. Despite wide variations, largely reflecting the constitution of the study populations, most authors have reported exercise echocardiography to be sensitive – identifying 80 to 85% of patients with significant coronary artery disease. Most studies have shown false positive rates of 10 to 15%, giving specificities in the 85 to 90% range. These results for specificity may be colored by the population undergoing

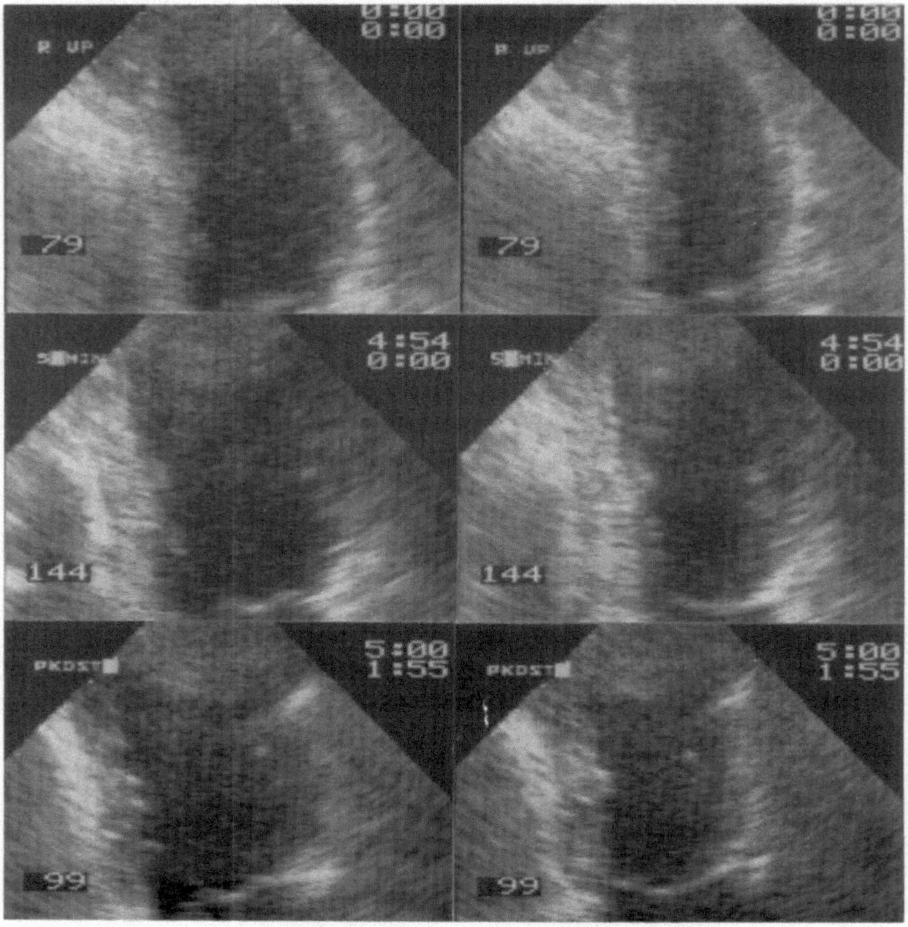

Figure 3.2. Diastolic (left) and systolic (right) images and traced outlines of the apical two-chamber view at rest, peak- and post-exercise showing rapid resolution of ischemia after bicycle stress. Contraction is homogeneous at rest (A), with an area of apical akinesia (arrows) at peak

angiography for symptoms suggestive of coronary disease – who may not, therefore, have normal hearts. Cardiomyopathic or microvascular processes may account for some abnormalities witnessed in this group, and normalcy rates (reflecting the results of the test in a population with a low probability of coronary disease) are an alternative method of assessing the ability of the test to identify normal myocardium. Two studies have reported normalcy rates of over 90% [5,30].

Table 3.1 also illustrates the long history of this technique, showing that its wider adoption has correlated with improvements in equipment and image

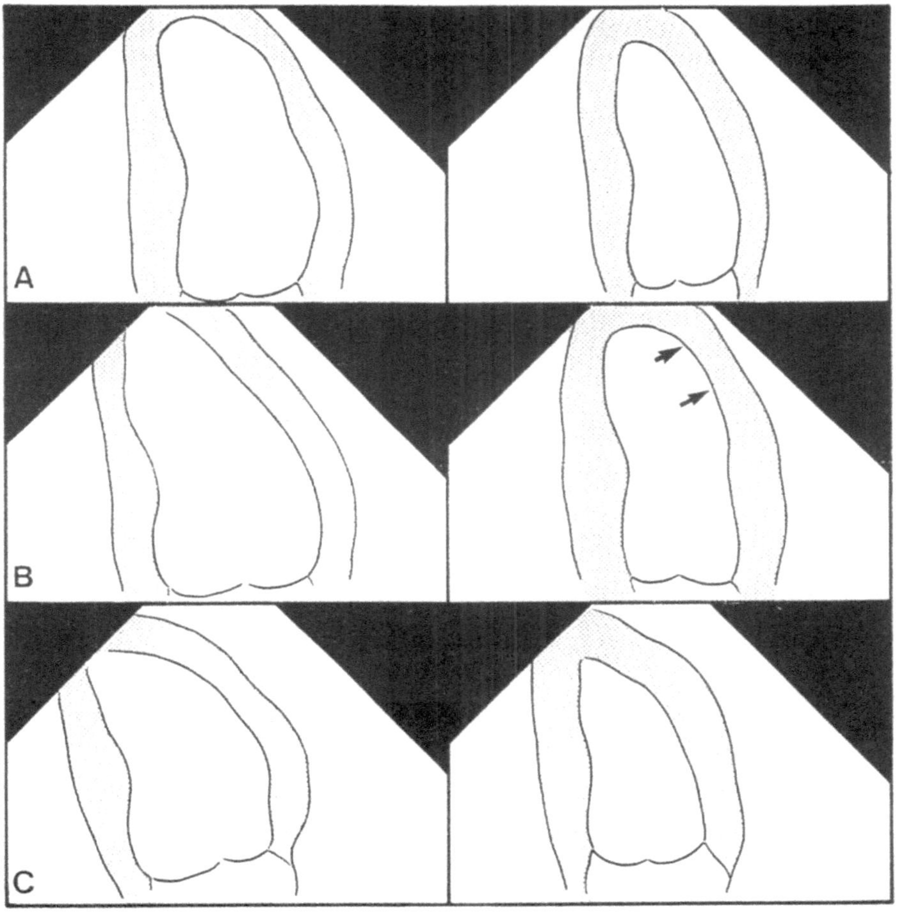

stress (B), with normal function one minute post-exercise (C). The patient had a mild (60%) stenosis of the left anterior descending coronary artery.

digitization over the last 7 years. Interestingly, despite the facilitation of the technique by digital acquisition and review [35], the benefits of digitization are not apparent as an enhancement of accuracy. However, direct comparison of blinded results using digital and video play-back in the same patients has suggested an increment of sensitivity with the use of image digitization, for both exercise and non-exercise techniques (TM, unpublished data).

Several methodologic and clinical aspects influence the reported accuracy of exercise echocardiography. The methodologic influences include; a) the definition of coronary stenosis significance, b) exclusion of patients with technically difficult studies, and c) the type of stress. Patient parameters

Table 3.1. Sensitivity and specificity of exercise echocardiography for the diagnosis of coronary arter

Author	Year	Ref	n	Stress technique	Success rate	CAD deftn	Multivessel (% all CAD)	MI (% all CAD
Wann	79	14	28	SB	71%	>50%	13 (87%)	8 (53%)
Morganroth	81	15	55	SB	78%	>50%	25 (78%)	18 (56%)
Maurer	81	16	48	TM	85%	>50%	17 (74%)	0
Visser	83	17	52	SB	75%	>50%	15 (58%)	6 (23%)
Limacher	83	18	73	TM	100%	>50%	45 (80%)	33 (59%)
Robertson	83	10	30	TM	92%	>75%	13 (62%)	14 (67%)
Ginzton	84	19	41	UB	95%	MI	–	23 (100%)
Armstrong	86	20	95	TM, D	100%	>50%	45 (56%)	36 (45%)
Armstrong	87	21	123	TM, D	–	>50%	59 (58%)	50 (50%)
Ryan	88	22	64	TM, D	–	>50%	15 (38%)	0
Voelker	88	23	56	SB	86%	>50%	22 (65%)	19 (56%)
Sawada	89	24	57	TM/UB, D	100%	>50%	11 (39%)	0
Sheikh	90	25	34	TM, D	–	>50%	0	0
Crouse	91	26	228	TM, D	–	>50%	106 (61%)	–
Mertes	91	27	150	SB, D	90%	–	–	–
Agati	91	28	57	SB, D	–	>85%	0	–
Galanti	91	29	53	UB, D	–	>70%	14 (48%)	0
Marwick	92	30	150	TM, D	100%	>50%	54 (47%)	55 (48%)
Pozzoli	92	31	75	UB, D	–	>50%	16 (33%)	0
Salustri	92	32	44	UB, D	–	>50%	0	0
Quinones	92	33	112	TM, D	–	>50%	45 (52%)	–
Hecht	93	5	180	SB, D	100%	>50%	82 (60%)	38 (28%)
Ryan	93	34	309	UB, D	100%	>50%	126 (60%)	132 (63%)

CAD = coronary artery disease, CAD defntn = stenosis diameter for definition of CAD, D = image digi angiography, ref = reference number, RV = right ventricle, SB = supine bicycle, SVD = single vess

influencing test results include; i) previous myocardial infarction, ii) the extent and severity of coronary disease, and iii) the site of coronary disease.

3.2.1 *Methodologic Influences on the Accuracy of Exercise Echocardiography*

a. Definition of Stenosis Significance. Coronary stenoses occur in a spectrum of severity, but for studies of accuracy, an arbitrary cutoff must be assigned to define "significant" disease. Use of > 50% diameter stenosis (the most common cutoff) identifies almost all lesions limiting flow under conditions of peak vasodilation, but also includes some stenoses which are physiologically non-significant – use of this standard may thus limit sensitivity but is associated with high specificity. Conversely, use of a > 70% cutoff ensures that practically all "significant" stenoses are flow-limiting (hence producing a high sensitivity), but some stenoses of < 70% diameter, despite classifica-

disease.

Sensitivity – overall	Sensitivity – SVD pts	Sensitivity MI excluded	Specificity	Comments
87% (n = 15)	50% (n = 2)	71% (n = 7)	100% (n = 5)	30 degree sector scan
66% (n = 32)	57% (n = 7)	57% (n = 21)	91% (n = 11)	
86% (n = 28)	50% (n = 6)	83% (n = 23)	69% (n = 13)	RV analyzed
77% (n = 26)	73% (n = 11)	70% (n = 20)	92% (n = 13)	30 degree sector scan
91% (n = 56)	64% (n = 11)	79% (n = 24)	88% (n = 17)	
100% (n = 21)	100% (n = 8)	100% (n = 7)	75% (n = 4)	On treatment
100% (n = 23)	–	–	100% (n = 16)	
88% (n = 80)	–	80% (n = 44)	87% (n = 15)	On treatment
88% (n = 101)	81% (n = 42)	78% (n = 51)	86% (n = 22)	
78% (n = 40)	76% (n = 25)	78% (n = 40)	100% (n = 24)	
41% (n = 34)	–	–	100% (n = 6)	Apical views only
86% (n = 28)	88% (n = 17)	86% (n = 28)	86% (n = 29)	Females only
81% (n = 21)	81% (n = 21)	81% (n = 21)	92% (n = 13)	Quant angio, max stress
97% (n = 175)	92% (n = 66)	–	64% (n = 53)	Normal = hypercontractile
87% (n = 121)	85% (n = 50)	–	80% (n = 29)	Apical imaging
81% (n = 27)	81% (n = 27)	81% (n = 27)	63% (n = 30)	Quant angio, max stress
93% (n = 27)	93% (n = 14)	93% (n = 27)	92% (n = 26)	
84% (n = 114)	77% (n = 60)	80% (n = 59)	86% (n = 36)	
71% (n = 49)	60% (n = 33)	71% (n = 49)	88% (n = 26)	
86% (n = 30)	86% (n = 30)	86% (n = 30)	64% (n = 14)	
74% (n = 86)	58% (n = 41)	–	81% (n = 26)	
93% (n = 137)	84% (n = 55)	100% (n = 82)	86% (n = 43)	
91% (n = 211)	86% (n = 85)	95% (n = 126)	78% (n = 98)	

zation, Echo = exercise echocardiogram, MI = myocardial infarction, quant angio = quantitative disease, TM = treadmill, UB = upright bicycle.

tion as "non-significant", are indeed physiologically important and compromise the measured specificity. Thus, using a > 75% stenosis cutoff, Robertson [10] reported a sensitivity of 100%, but a specificity of only 75%. Moreover, the qualitative interpretation of coronary arteriography as this "gold standard" is limited by observer variability [36], difficulties in assessing eccentric stenoses, and poor correlation between the anatomic severity of stenoses and their effects on flow [37,38]. Quantitative coronary arteriography [39] has circumvented some of these technical problems, with improved correlation with functional parameters [40]. Using quantitative angiography, Shiekh [25] found that a stenosis diameter of 50% gave a sensitivity of 81%, and a specificity of 92%. In that study, patients with single-vessel coronary disease developing wall motion abnormalities after maximal exercise had an absolute stenosis diameter of 1.0 mm, compared with 1.7 mm in those with visually assessed stenoses > 50% but without inducible ischemia. Using quantitative wall motion evaluation but an otherwise similar study design, Agati [28] found that the best correlate of abnormal function was an absolute lumen diameter of 0.7 mm, corresponding to an 85% stenosis diameter. The discrepancy between these studies may reflect the use of quantitative echocardiography in Agati's study, which requires a reduction of normal function for the diagnosis of ischemia (rather than inhomogeneity of contraction, which may be more sensitive).

b. Influence of Echocardiographic Image Quality. Although over 90 to 95% of images are usually interpretable, the quality of stress echocardiograms obviously varies from patient to patient. Studies which exclude technically poor quality examinations may enhance the apparent accuracy of the test, at the risk of making the data less relevant to routine practice. Recent reports involving unselected groups have also circumvented criticisms related to clinical applicability [20,24,30]. Regrettably, the influence of image quality on accuracy is difficult to measure. We devised a four-point subjective rating system for this purpose; an "A quality" study was defined by good endocardial definition, with good image quality in all views, "B quality" by images lacking endocardial definition, and/or failure to demonstrate wall motion in all views (as long as segments could be analysed in at least one view), "C quality" by failure to image all segments even in multiple views (but with all coronary territories visualized at least in part), and "D quality" defined by severely compromised images, with failure to visualize one or more coronary territories. We attempted to interpret all visualized segments, classifying all other regions as normal. In this study, suboptimal images (C and D quality) were not identified as predictive of sensitivity [30] because even in these instances, enough of the myocardium was apparent to permit visualization of the ischemic segments.

c. Influence of Stress Modality. Accuracy may be influenced by the type of stress used in so far that it must be sufficient to provoke ischemia. Handgrip stress [41] offers only a small increase in cardiac work, and is relatively insensitive: if patients cannot exercise with their legs, pharmacologic testing is preferable. Despite the theoretical advantages and disadvantages of treadmill and bicycle stress, recent results have been very similar with each. Combining data from multiple studies shows post-treadmill echocardiography [26,30,33] to have a sensitivity of 88% and specificity of 75%, compared with 88% and 77% for upright bicycle [29,31,32,34], and 90% and 80% for supine bicycle echocardiography [5,28]. Direct comparisons will be needed in large numbers of patients in order to determine whether any modality is superior.

3.2.2 *Clinical Influences on the Accuracy of Stress Echocardiography*

i) Myocardial Infarction. As echocardiography readily identifies the presence and site of prior infarction [42]; the inclusion of post-infarction patients inflates the sensitivity of exercise echocardiography for the identification of coronary artery disease. Moreover, the presence of coronary artery disease is usually already known from pre-test data in patients undergoing exercise testing after infarction; it is therefore inappropriate to include them in studies pertaining to the diagnosis of coronary artery disease. Thus, if patients are stratified according to presence or absence of electrocardiographic Q-waves [21], the sensitivity of a resting or stress-induced wall motion abnormality for the prediction of coronary disease among those with Q-wave evidence of prior infarction (98%) exceeds that in those without previous infarction (78%). The other approach used to avoid inflating the recorded levels of sensitivity with post-infarction patients is to exclude those with resting wall motion abnormalities. This also identifies lower levels of sensitivity [22], but may be excessively stringent, as it excludes individuals with severe chronic ischemia ("hibernation") and/or post-ischemic dysfunction ("stunning") without infarction [43]. Moreover, from a clinical perspective, stratification on the basis of a resting wall motion abnormality is less sound, as this may only be known if the patient has already had a resting echocardiogram – implying the inclusion of this test to the diagnostic sequence. For these reasons, in our own work, "infarction" is defined by Q-wave criteria.

While inclusion of post-infarction patients in studies of overall diagnostic accuracy is inappropriate, stress echocardiography still has a role in this group. As discussed in later chapters, the clinical question in these circumstances pertains not to the diagnosis of coronary disease, but to the ability to identify heterozonal ischemia (or "ischemia at a distance"), homozonal ischemia (or peri-infarct ischemia), and myocardial viability. The detection of coronary disease by stress echocardiography in a territory other than that of the infarct-related artery is reported to range from 65% [21] to 72% [30] – a range comparable to the results of thallium scintigraphy in the equivalent situation. While stunned (viable) myocardium has been shown to be responsive to sympathomimetic agents [44], the role of the sympathomimetic effects of exercise in this respect is unknown. In practice, subtle changes in pre-existing wall motion abnormalities are difficult enough to identify in a resting patient during dobutamine stress, and may be impossible under the more difficult circumstances of exercise stress.

ii) Coronary Disease Extent and Severity. Patients with significant stenoses in one or more coronary vessels are likely to have a larger area of ischemic myocardium. The implications of this are a larger area of abnormal wall motion and/or a more severe wall motion abnormality. Indeed, while collateral flow may protect a region with single vessel disease, this cannot occur in situations where collateral vessels are themselves compromised by stenoses. Not surprisingly, many studies (Table 3.1) have shown the sensitivity of exercise echocardiography to be lower in the presence of single vessel disease. However, the sensitivity of exercise echocardiography for single vessel disease has varied form 76 to 93% in recent studies of digital echocardiography [26–34]. This variation is caused by modulation of the effect of single vessel disease by other factors, so that ischemia may be induced notwithstanding the presence of single vessel disease if lesions are severe or proximal.

Increasing stenosis severity has a similar effect. Milder stenoses, even if they limit peak hyperemic flow, may produce little or no ischemia. In Sheikh's study of quantitative angiography and exercise echocardiography, only about half of a group of patients with 50–70% stenoses demonstrated echocardiographic evidence of ischemia [25]. In our experience, the angiographic predictors of false negative results were shown to be the presence of single vessel and mild coronary disease [30]. Fortunately, the group of patients with negative stress echocardiograms have a relatively benign prognosis [45].

iii) Site of Coronary Disease. Ischemia involving the posterior wall of the left ventricle is potentially difficult to detect with ECG or nuclear perfusion imaging. The same does not appear to be true of stress echocardiography. In our experience of detection of single-vessel coronary disease [30], 77% of 26 left anterior descending and 69% of 26 right or circumflex stenoses were identified. In a stepwise logistic regression model, Armstrong [21] reported that proximal left anterior descending and circumflex lesions were independently associated with the presence of an abnormal exercise echocardiogram. The ability of stress echocardiography to recognise the presence of disease in individual vessels is discussed further, below.

iv) Exercise Capacity. In patients with chronic stable angina, myocardial ischemia becomes apparent after the oxygen requirements of the heart are increased, and exceed the ability of the coronary arteries to increase perfusion. Thus, the sensitivity of the exercise ECG, stress thallium imaging and nuclear ventriculography are all compromised by the performance of submaximal exercise [46–48]. The results of post-treadmill stress echocardiography are influenced in the same way [30], with 39% of false negative results reflecting the performance of submaximal stress, defined by failure to achieve 85% of age-predicted maximal heart-rate. In accordance with the lower heart-rate response of bicycle exercise, the influence of this variable is less prominent – both Hecht [5] and Ryan [34] have shown failure to achieve target heart-rate is not predictive of false negative scans in this setting.

3.3 Causes of False Negative and False Positive Exercise Echocardiogram Results

Assessment of the accuracy of exercise echocardiography is based upon the comparison of anatomic (angiographic) and functional (echocardiographic) indices of coronary disease. Unfortunately, the binary distinction between disease being "present" or "absent" requires an arbitrary separation, the level of which influences values for sensitivity and specificity, as described

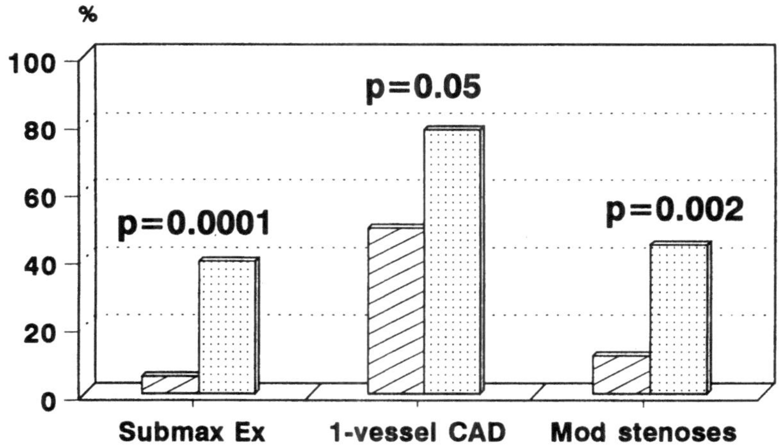

	Submax Ex	1-vessel CAD	Mod stenoses
EE correct	5	49	11
EE incorrect	39	78	44

Figure 3.3. Frequency of single vessel disease, moderate (50–70%) coronary stenoses, and submaximal exercise among patients with incorrect (false negative) and correct (true positive) stress echocardiograms.

above. Some "inaccuracies" merely reflect these limitations, for example, a "false negative" stress echocardiogram in the presence of a "significant" 60% stenosis may be due to the absence of ischemia engendered by this lesion rather than any shortcoming of the test itself. In summary, there is no perfect "gold standard" for judging the presence of significant coronary disease.

Nonetheless, not all inaccuracies are due to the problems inherent in the comparison of anatomic and functional tests. Milder grades of coronary disease (moderate stenoses especially in a single vessel), although limiting flow, may induce small regions of ischemia that are not identifiable by stress echocardiography. Other causes of false negative results include poor image quality, delayed post-exercise imaging, continued anti-anginal medications and submaximal exercise [30]. The latter three of these occur because ischemia resolves before imaging or does not occur at all (Figure 3.3). In these situations, use of the term "non-diagnostic" should be considered for reporting negative test results.

The causes of false positive stress echocardiograms are less well understood than for false negative studies, but potentially reflect methodologic and patient-related problems. False positive results are likely if mild abnormalities are over-interpreted, especially in the context of suboptimal (especially off-axis) views. A specific problem in this respect pertains to the basal inferior wall, which may be partially shadowed by the papillary muscle in the apical 2–chamber view, as well as being tethered to the adjacent valve ring. Our practice is to be particularly circumspect in the interpretation of wall motion abnormalities restricted to this area alone; unless abnormal wall motion is demonstrated in another view and/or in an adjacent segment, we err on the side of being conservative in the identification of ischemia at this site. Patient-related false positives may arise if patients with non-coronary heart disease are included – not all stress-induced abnormalities of global left ventricular function are due to ischemia. Indeed, in active individuals, lack of hyperkinesia and overt hypokinesia may occur after maximal stress, suggesting that such persons may require the application of different criteria to most other patients undergoing stress echocardiography [49]. Moreover, studies with stress nuclear ventriculography in patients with valvular regurgitation have suggested that apparent regional wall motion abnormalities may also be detected [50]. Whether this is also true of stress echocardiography remains to be defined.

3.4 Identification of Stenoses in Individual Coronary Vessels

The ability of exercise echocardiography to detect coronary disease does not appear to be influenced by its site. Moreover, several studies have indicated that the test is able to accurately identify the lesion responsible for ischemia. Such analyses have been based upon standardized models for the prediction of vascular territories supplied by each vessel (see Chapter 2), whereby the septal, anteroseptal, anterior and apical walls are ascribed to the left anterior descending, the posterior and lateral walls to the left circumflex, and the inferior and inferoseptal walls to the right coronary artery. Of course, this scheme is a generalization of the findings in individual patients, where the vascular territories are highly variable. The commonest source of ambiguity is the posterior wall (supplied by either right or circumflex coronary artery, depending on their relative size), and some authors have compensated for this by combining the right and circumflex systems into a common, posterior system. In our experience of locating the site of pathology in patients with single-vessel disease, regional sensitivities were 77% for the anterior descending, 67% for the circumflex, and 70% for the right coronary [30]. In an entire study group (including patients with multivessel disease and previous infarction), Hecht reported respective sensitivities of 95%, 78% and 81% [5]. However, Armstrong [21] predicted left circumflex disease correctly in only 22% of patients with stenoses in this vessel, and Pozzoli [31] reported a sensitivity of 45% for recognition of left circumflex disease as such. The source of this variation is unclear – in addition to the variation in coronary anatomy, it may reflect problems with resolution of the lateral wall endocardium because of the parallel orientation of the wall and ultrasound beam,

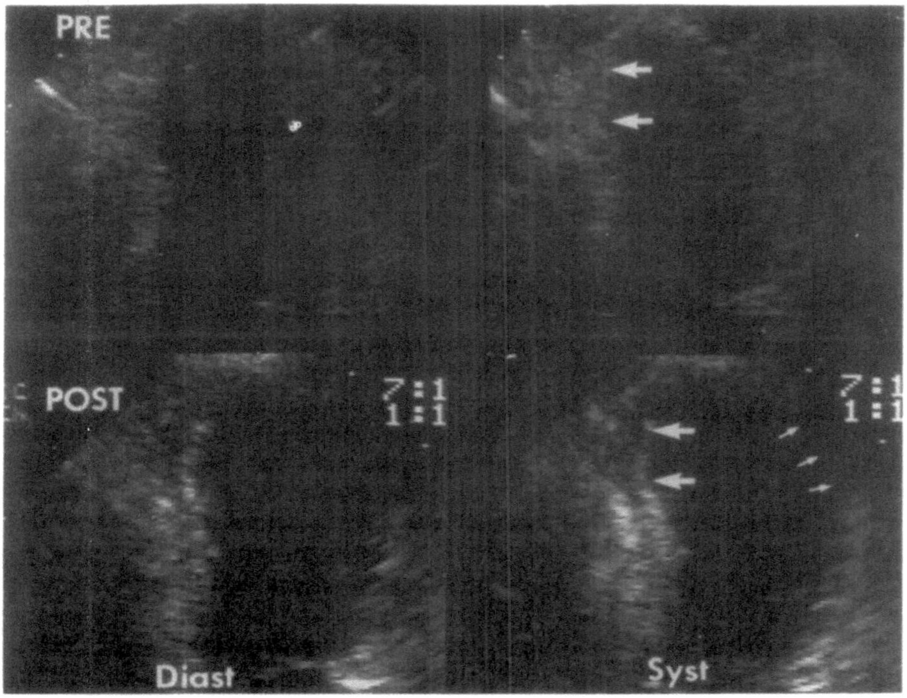

Figure 3.4. Identification of multivessel coronary disease in a patient with a previous myocardial infarction. A resting wall motion abnormality is identified (large arrow) in the distal septum, reflecting prior infarction in the territory of the left anterior descending coronary artery. Exercise-induced regional dysfunction, due to left circumflex stenosis, is apparent in the lateral wall. Reproduced with permission of the Journal of the American College of Cardiology.

and problems of lateral resolution. The circumflex territory may also be small in some patients.

3.5 Diagnosis of Multivessel Disease by Exercise Echocardiography

Exercise echocardiography more readily identifies myocardial ischemia in the setting of multivessel disease. A different aspect relates to the ability of this test to recognise multivessel disease as such (Figures 3.4 and 3.5). Again, these analyses are colored by the application of assumptions relating to the relative distributions of the coronary arteries. The accuracy of stress echocardiography for the recognition of multivessel disease differs in patients with and without resting wall motion abnormalities due to myocardial infarction.

Multivessel disease is readily recognized in patients with previous myocardial infarction. In an unselected group [30], 88% of patients with multivessel disease who were able to perform maximal exercise showed "ischemia at a distance". These results reflect the fact that the presence of a resting wall motion abnormality effectively defines the presence of disease in one territory, so that ischemia need occur in only one region for the coronary anatomy to be predicted. The situation of patients without previous infarction is quite different, in that two or more regions must become ischemic for multivessel disease to be predicted. In this context, ischemia in one zone may limit exercise before the cardiac workload is enough to precipitate ischemia in another less severely diseased area. In addition, the examiner's eye tends to concentrate on the most severely ischemic region, as the test centers upon the comparitive interpretation of segments with each other. These features may explain the lower sensitivity of stress echocardiography for the prediction

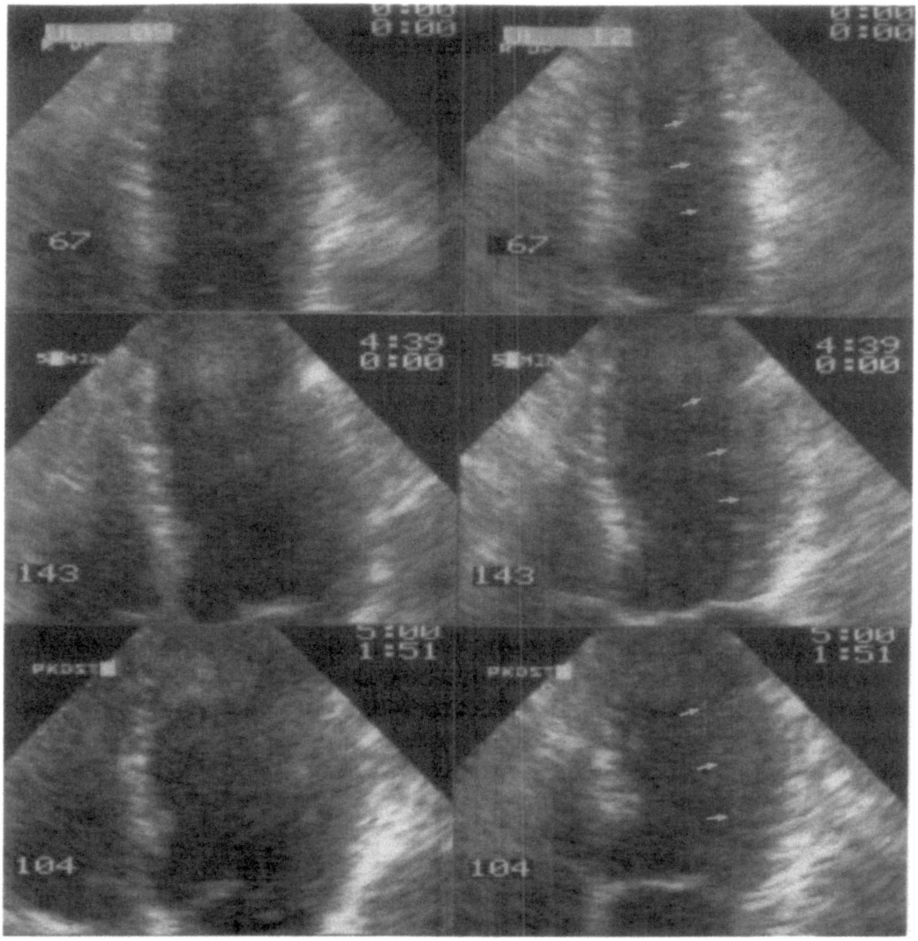

Figure 3.5. Identification of multivessel coronary disease in a patient without previous myocardial infarction. At rest (top) the septum and lateral walls contract homogeneously. At peak exercise, the septum is thinned and akinetic, and the lateral wall is hypokinetic (arrows). After exercise, the proximal septum recovers, but the apex does not, and the lateral wall, although thickening more, has not returned to normal.

to age, gender, medical therapy, number of diseased vessels, and exercise parameters, no differences in the extent or severity of ischemia were apparent between the 48 patients with silent ischemia and the remaining 26 with angina. This study exemplifies the benefits of stress echocardiography with respect to visualizing disease extent (because of its high-resolution tomographic imaging) and severity (because of the ability to score regional function).

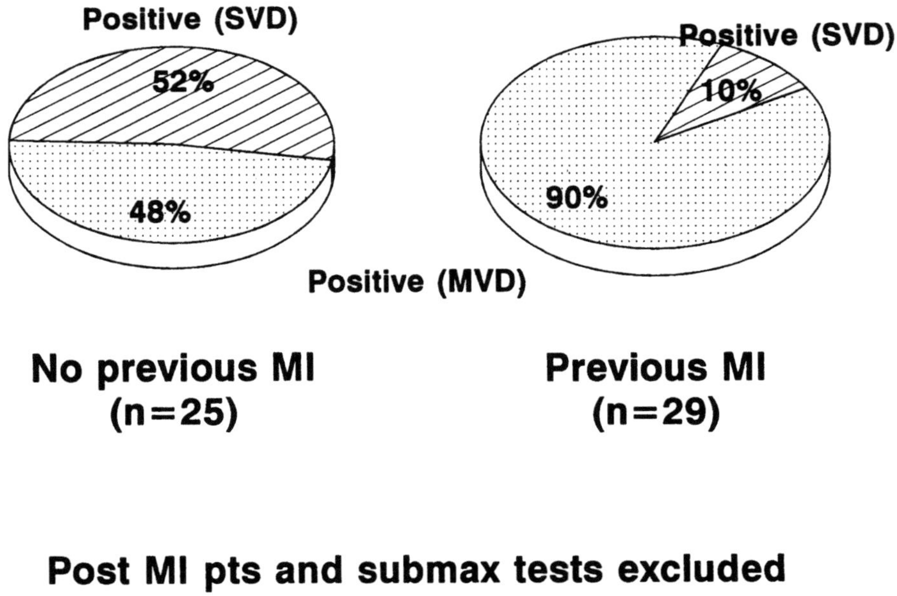

Figure 3.6. Recognition of multivessel disease in patients with and without previous myocardial infarction [30].

3.6 Conclusion

Exercise echocardiography has become accepted as a feasible technique for the identification of coronary artery disease. Treadmill and bicycle stress are equally applicable, and the selection of one or other technique should reflect the locally preferred stress methodology, as well as the patient's ability to use either device.

The test is generally accurate for the detection of coronary disease, as well as its site. Situations associated with an increased probability of false negative results have been characterized, and in circumstances where such test factors (eg submaximal stress) are present in conjunction with a negative result, the test should be reported as non-diagnostic, rather than negative. Likewise, the ability of the test to identify the absence of multivessel disease in patients without previous infarction is limited.

References

1. Feigenbaum H. Exercise echocardiography. J Am Soc Echo 1988;1:161–6.
2. Marwick T, Stewart WJ, Salcedo EE. Exercise echocardiographic and Doppler evaluation of left ventricular function. Am J Card Imaging 1991;5:281–90.
3. Presti CF, Armstrong WF, Feigenbaum H. Comparison of echocardiography at peak exerc-

ise and after bicycle exercise in evaluation of patients with known or suspected coronary artery disease. J Am Soc Echo 1988;1:119–26.
4. Ginzton LE. Stress echocardiography and myocardial contrast echocardiography. Cardiol Clin 1989;7:493–509.
5. Hecht HS, DeBord L, Shaw R *et al.* Digital supine bicycle stress echocardiography: A new technique for evaluating coronary artery disease. J Am Coll Cardiol 1993;21:950–6.
6. Heng MK, Simard M, Lake R, Udhoji VH. Exercise two-dimensional echocardiography for diagnosis of coronary artery disease. Am J Cardiol 1984;54:502–7.
7. Astrand PO, Saltin B. Maximum oxygen uptake and heart-rate in various types of muscular activity. J Appl Physiol 1961;16:977–81.
8. Niederberger M, Bruce RA, Kusumi F, Whitkanack S. Disparities in ventilatory and circulatory responses to bicycle and treadmill exercise. Br Heart J 1974;36:377–82.
9. Currie PJ, Kelly MJ, Pitt A. Comparison of supine and erect bicycle exercise electrocardiography in coronary heart disease: accentuation of exercise-induced ischemic ST depression by supine position. Am J Cardiol 1983;52:1167–73.
10. Robertson WS, Feigenbaum H, Armstrong WF, Dillon JC, O'Donnell J, McHenry PW. Exercise echocardiography: A clinically practical addition in the evaluation of coronary artery disease. J Am Coll Cardiol 1983;2:1085–91.
11. Dymond DS, Foster C, Greiner RP, Carpenter J, Schmidt DH. Peak exercise and immediate post-exercise imaging for the detection of left ventricular functional abnormalities in coronary artery disease. Am J Cardiol 1984;53:1532–7.
12. Applegate RJ, Dell'Italia LJ, Crawford MH. Usefulness of two-dimensional echocardiography during low-level exercise testing early after uncomplicated myocardial infarction. Am J Cardiol 1987;60:10–4.
13. Bairey CN, Rozanski A, Berman DS. Exercise echocardiography: Ready or not? J Am Coll Cardiol 1988;11:1355–8.
14. Wann S, Faris J, Childress R, Dillon J, Weyman A, Feigenbaum H. Exercise cross-sectional echocardiography in ischemic heart disease. Circulation 1979;60:1300–8.
15. Morganroth J, Chen CC, David D *et al.* Exercise cross-sectional echocardiographic diagnosis of coronary artery disease. Am J Cardiol 1981;47:20–6.
16. Maurer G, Nanda NC. Two dimensional echocardiographic evaluation of exercise-induced left and right ventricular asynergy: Correlation with thallium scanning. Am J Cardiol 1981;48:720–7.
17. Visser CA, van der Wieken RL, Kan G *et al.* Comparison of two-dimensional echocardiography with radionuclide angiography during dynamic exercise for the detection of coronary artery disease. Am Heart J 1983;106:528–34.
18. Limacher MC, Quinones MA, Poliner LR, Nelson JG, Winters WL, Waggoner AD. Detection of coronary artery disease with exercise two-dimensional echocardiography: Description of a clinically applicable method and comparison with radionuclide ventriculography. Circulation 1983;67:1211–8.
19. Ginzton LE, Conant R, Brizendine M, Lee F, Mena I, Laks M. Exercise subcostal two-dimensional echocardiography: A new method of segmental wall motion abnormality. Am J Cardiol 1984;53:805–11.
20. Armstrong WF, O'Donnell J, Dillon JC, McHenry PL, Morris SN, Feigenbaum H. Complementary value of two-dimensional exercise echocardiography to routine treadmill testing. Ann Intern Med 1986;105:829–35.
21. Armstrong WF, O'Donnell J, Ryan T, Feigenbaum H. Effect of prior myocardial infarction and extent and location of coronary disease on accuracy of exercise echocardiography. J Am Coll Cardiol 1987;10:531–8.
22. Ryan T, Vasey CG, Presti CF, O'Donnell J, Feigenbaum H, Armstrong WF. Exercise echocardiography: Detection of coronary artery disease in patients with normal left ventricular wall motion at rest. J Am Coll Cardiol 1988;11:993–9.
23. Voelker W, Jacksch R, Dittman H, Karsch KR. Diagnostic accuracy of 2–D echocardiography for detection of exercise-induced wall motion abnormalities in patients with coronary

artery disease: Comparison with biplane cineventriculography. Clin Cardiol 1988;11:547–52.

24. Sawada SG, Ryan T, Fineberg NS *et al.* Exercise echocardiographic detection of coronary artery disease in women. J Am Coll Cardiol 1989;14:1440–7.
25. Sheikh KH, Bengtson JR, Helmy S *et al.* Relation of quantitative coronary lesion measurements to the development of exercise-induced ischemia assessed by exercise echocardiography. J Am Coll Cardiol 1990;15:1043–51.
26. Crouse LJ, Harbrecht JJ, Vacek JL, Rosamond TL, Kramer PH. Exercise echocardiography as a screening test for coronary artery disease and correlation with angiography. Am J Cardiol 1991;67:1213–8.
27. Mertes H, Erbel R, Nixdorff U, Mohr-Kahaly S, Wolfinger D, Meyer J. Stress echocardiography: A sensitive method for the detection of coronary artery disease. Herz 1991;16:355–66.
28. Agati L, Arata L, Luongo R *et al.* Assessment of severity of coronary narrowings by quantitative exercise echocardiography and comparison with quantitative arteriography. Am J Cardiol 1991;67:1201–7.
29. Galanti G, Sciagra R, Comeglio M *et al.* Diagnostic accuracy of peak exercise echocardiography in coronary artery disease: Comparison with thallium-201 myocardial scintigraphy. Am Heart J 1991;122:1609–16.
30. Marwick T, Nemec J, Pashkow F, Stewart WJ, Salcedo E. Accuracy and limitations of exercise echocardiography in a routine clinical setting. J Am Coll Cardiol 1992;19:74–81.
31. Pozzoli MM, Fioretti PM, Salustri A, Reijs AE, Roelandt JR. Exercise echocardiography and technetium-99 m MIBI single photon emission computed tomography in the detection of coronary artery disease. Am J Cardiol 1991;67:350–5.
32. Salustri A, Pozzoli MM, Hermans W *et al.* Relationship between exercise echocardiography and perfusion single photon emission computed tomography in patients with single vessel coronary artery disease. Am Heart J 1992;124:75–83.
33. Quinones MA, Verani MS, Haichin RM, Mahmarian JJ, Suarez J, Zoghbi WA. Exercise echocardiography versus Tl-201 single photon emission computed tomography in evaluation of coronary artery disease. Analysis of 292 patients. Circulation 1992;85:1026–31.
34. Ryan T, Segar DS, Sawada SG *et al.* Detection of coronary artery disease with upright bicycle exercise echocardiography. J Am Soc Echocardiogr 1993;6:186–97.
35. West SR, Feigenbaum H, Armstrong WF, Green D, Dillon JC. Split screen simultaneous digital imaging of rest and stress echocardiograms – A new method for evaluation of exercise-induced wall motion abnormalities [abstract]. J Am Coll Cardiol 1984;3:563.
36. Zir LM, Miller SW, Dinsmore RE, Gilbert JP, Harthorne JW. Interobserver variability in coronary angiography. Circulation 1976;53:627–32.
37. White CW, Wright CB, Doty DB *et al.* Does visual interpretation of the coronary arteriogram predict the physiologic importance of a coronary stenosis? N Engl J Med 1984;310:819–24.
38. Rosenberg MC, Klein LW, Agarwal JB, Stets G, Hermann GA, Helfant RH. Quantification of absolute luminal diameter by computer analyzed digital subtraction angiography: An assessment in human coronary arteries. Circulation 1988;77:484–9.
39. Zylstra F, van Ommeren J, Reiber JH, Serruys PW. Does the quantitative assessment of coronary artery dimensions predict the physiologic significance of a coronary stenosis? Circulation 1987;75:1154–61.
40. Marcus M, Skorton DJ, Johnson MR, Collins SM, Harrison DG, Kerber RE. Visual estimates of percent diameter coronary stenosis: "A battered gold standard". J Am Coll Cardiol 1988;11:882–5.
41. Mitamura H, Ogawa S, Hori S *et al.* Two-dimensional echocardiographic analysis of wall motion abnormalities during handgrip exercise in patients with coronary artery disease. Am J Cardiol 1981;48:711–9.
42. Corday E, Hajduczki I, O'Byrne GT, Kar S, Areeda J, Corday SR. Echocardiographic

criteria to distinguish reversible from irreversible myocardial ischaemia. Eur Heart J 1988;9(Suppl F):29–43.

43. Kloner RA, Przyklenk K, Patel B. Altered myocardial states: The stunned and hibernating myocardium. Am J Med 1986;86(Suppl 1A):14–21.
44. Ellis SG, Wynne J, Braunwald E, Henschke CI, Sandor T, Kloner RA. Response of reperfusion-salvaged, stunned myocardium to inotropic stimulation. Am Heart J 1984;107:13–9.
45. Sawada SG, Ryan T, Conley MJ, Corya BC, Feigenbaum H, Armstrong WF. Prognostic value of a normal exercise echocardiogram. Am Heart J 1990;120:49–55.
46. Cumming GR. Yield of ischemic exercise electrocardiograms in relation to exercise intensity in a normal population. Br Heart J 1972;34:919–23.
47. Brady TJ, Thrall JH, Lo K, Pitt B. The importance of adequate exercise in the detection of coronary heart disease by radionuclide ventriculography. J Nucl Med 1980;21:1125–30.
48. Iskandrian AS, Heo J, Kong B, Lyons E. Effect of exercise level on the ability of thallium-201 tomographic imaging in detecting coronary artery disease: Analysis of 461 patients. J Am Coll Cardiol 1989;14:1477–86.
49. Fisman EZ, Frank AG, Ben-Ari E *et al.* Altered left ventricular volume and ejection fraction responses to supine dynamic exercise in athletes. J Am Coll Cardiol 1990;15:582–8.
50. Hecht HS, Hopkins JM, Exercise induced regional wall motion abnormalities on radionuclide angiography: Lack of reliability for detection of coronary artery disease in the presence of valvular heart disease. Am J Cardiol 1981;47:861–6.
51. Marwick T, Nemec J, Torelli J, Salcedo EE, Stewart WJ. Extent and severity of abnormal left ventricular wall motion detected by exercise echocardiography during painful and silent ischemia. Am J Cardiol 1992;69:1483–4.
52. Cohn RF, Brown EJ, Wynne J, Holman L, Atkins HA. Global and regional left ventricular ejection fraction abnormalities during exercise in patients with silent myocardial ischemia. J Am Coll Cardiol 1983;1:931–3.
53. Vassiliadis IV, Machac J, O'Hara M, Sezhiyan T, Horowitz SF. Exercise-induced myocardial dysfunction in patients with coronary artery disease with and without angina. Am Heart J 1991;121:1403–8.

4. Stress Echocardiography Using Exercise-Simulating Techniques

The choice of techniques for inducing ischemia at stress echocardiography corresponds to that for the scintigraphic methods, and involves a fundamental distinction between exercise and non-exercise approaches. The latter include exercise-simulating methods (including sympathomimetic and pacing stresses), which increase myocardial oxygen demand, and vasoactive agents (principally dipyridamole and ergonovine stresses), which primarily influence myocardial blood supply. This chapter will examine the exercise-simulating techniques, and explore whether their use is justifiable in preference to exercise stress. The following chapter will deal with the vasoactive stress agents.

4.1 Indications for Use of Exercise Simulating Agents

Pharmacologic and pacing stresses are usually reserved for patients who are unable to exercise. Stress echocardiography for the diagnosis of coronary artery disease in patients with peripheral vascular, orthopedic and neurologic limitations may mandate the use of a non-exercise stress. This may also be true for patients who are in a poor state of fitness, especially the elderly, in whom the test has been shown to be well tolerated and reliable [1]. Stress echocardiography may also be indicated for prognostic reasons in "at risk" patients undergoing operative treatment for vascular and orthopedic conditions where intervention may improve the functional state of the patient. In such circumstances, concerns relate not only to the avoidance of perioperative cardiac events, but also the prediction of occult coronary disease, which may become apparent after the operative treatment of non-cardiac exercise limitation (see Chapter 9).

Particular clinical circumstances may also favor the use of non-exercise stress. The performance of stress echocardiography in the cardiac catherization laboratory or the operating room may assist in clinical decision-making regarding the adequacy of revascularization. However, augmentation of oxygen demand by exercise is not possible in these situations, which necessitate the use of a non-exercise stress.

Finally, even in the routine stress laboratory, there are some attractions to the use of pharmacologic, in preference to exercise stress. Dobutamine

T.H. Marwick, Stress Echocardiography, 61–80.

stress may be particularly indicated for the detection of viable myocardium in patients with previous myocardial infarction (see Chapter 10). There is also some support for its widespread use instead of exercise, based upon advantages inherent in the nature of the stress and the imaging protocol. The incremental nature of the stress means that the time-course of ischemia may be identified – these data are not available using post-treadmill stress, and are more diificult to obtain at bicycle exercise. The imaging benefits of pharmacologic testing relate to the relative technical ease of image acquisition and better image quality inherent in (essentially) resting imaging – improvements which may permit the use of more quantitative reporting techniques. Indeed, the presumptive merits of pharmacologic stress echocardiography are analogous to those of stress thallium imaging with dipyridamole [2]. Similarly, the technical demands of performing peak- or post-exercise imaging have led to the advocation of non-exercise stressors for all patients.

4.2 Exercise Simulation Using Pharmacologic Stressors

4.2.1 *Pharmacologic Considerations*

The exercise simulating agents include dobutamine, dopamine, epinephrine and isopreterenol. As the name of the group suggests, their mechanism of action involves the induction of ischemia (and hence abnormal function) by increasing cardiac work and thereby oxygen requirements, in a fashion analogous to that of exercise. For this to be completely true, the myocardial metabolic effects of these agents should parallel changes in hemodynamics. In the case of dobutamine, however, experimental data [3] have suggested that there may be a metabolic stress additive to increased cardiac work (see Chapter 1). In addition, the sympathomimetic agents all cause a maldistribution of coronary flow, involving a dose-dependent reduction of subendocardial perfusion in the face of mild coronary stenoses [4]. This flow maldistribution does not appear to be the dominant source of ischemia, which instead reflects the development of tachycardia [5].

Despite the similarities between these agents, they are not interchangeable. Although epinephrine and isopreterenol have been used for stress testing [6,7], their arrhythmogenic consequences are clearly a disadvantage. Concern about these side-effects may limit the administered dose, compromising the degree of stress and thereby the sensitivity of the test (see below). Dopamine causes more alpha-stimulation and consequently may cause problems if it extravasates. It may also be less effective than dobutamine in terms of precipitating myocardial ischemia [8]. Dobutamine has become the most commonly administered exercise simulating agent, and the subsequent section is predominantly directed towards analysis of this pharmacologic stress. A derivative, arbutamine [9], also shows promise in this respect, but the relative benefits of this, compared with its parent compound, are ill-defined.

As dobutamine is predominantly a beta-1 agonist, its main initial effect is as an inotrope; this facilitates the detection of zones with abnormal function, as normal areas become hyperkinetic in response to the drug. Other receptors are stimulated to a lesser degree, so that vasodilation and chronotropy appear at higher doses [8,10], usually at the 20 mcg/kg/min level of the routine stress protocols. This chronotropic response, involving a mean heart-rate increment of 40 to 50 beats/minute and mean peak heart-rates of 110–120 beats/minute [11–17], appears to be the most important factor in terms of precipitating ischemia. Blood pressure normally rises, but may fall at higher doses, usually reflecting the vasodilator effects of this agent. Coronary flow in normal vessels is augmented by increasing myocardial oxygen demand, as well as a weak vasodilator effect. This aspect permits the combination of dobutamine stress with perfusion scintigraphy, which depicts regional variations in coronary flow reserve [18,19]. Finally, the half-life of dobutamine is so short (2–3 minutes) that complications or ischemia resolve promptly.

4.2.2 *Dobutamine Stress Protocol*

Patients are prepared for stress testing in the standard fashion; the test is performed in the fasting state, and patients are usually asked to stop anti-ischemic drugs on the day of the procedure. Chest lead monitoring may be modified (as in the case of exercise echocardiography) to remove electrodes from the echocardiographic windows, and intravenous access is secured. In addition to standard resuscitation equipment, intravenous beta-adrenoceptor blocking agents and nitrates should be available, in order to treat severe ischemia.

Dobutamine is usually administered incrementally, starting at 5 mcg/kg/min, and increasing to 40 mcg/kg/min in 2 or 3 minute stages [11–17]. The peak dose of 40 mcg/kg/min is now widely adopted, but variants include maximal doses of up to 50 mcg/kg/min and down to 20 mcg/kg/min [13,15]. Lower dose-rates administered over longer periods are able to attain similar hemodynamic effects to the high-dose protocols [15]; the relative plasma levels with different dose-regimens have not been studied. The standard dobutamine protocol has been combined with atropine in those in whom the test is negative at peak dose [20], and this maneuver is of particular benefit in patients on beta-blocking drugs. The addition of atropine produces a major increment of heart-rate and is effective in inducing ischemia. It appears to be safe, although there is less published experience than with standard dobutamine testing. Unfortunately, however, many non-diagnostic results at dobutamine testing reflect premature termination of the stress due to side-effects (see below), and the addition of atropine is unlikely to be of benefit in these situations.

The end-points of the test are completion of the protocol, development of severe angina or left ventricular dysfunction, or the development of intolerable side-effects. The patient is monitored continuously, using clinical

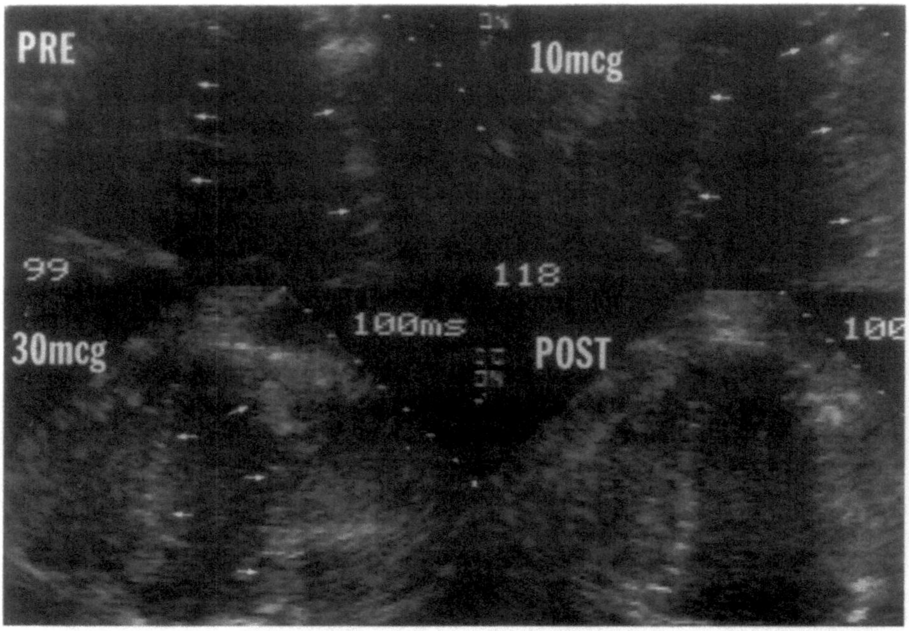

Figure 4.1. End-systolic images from a dobutamine echocardiogram, showing normal function at rest, little change at low-dose, hyperkinesis (arrows) at high-dose, and rapid resolution post-stress. Reproduced with permission of the American Journal of Cardiac Imaging.

signs, the electrocardiogram, and 2D-echocardiography (with storage on video-tape). Because only four digitized cine-loops can be displayed at once on the quad-screen display, we currently select a resting image, low-dose (10 mcg), and two high dose images, usually 30 and 40 mg. Other protocols involve digitization of rest, low-dose, high-dose and post-stress images (Figure 4.1). Other authors describe filling the quadrants with images at rest, at the first dose (5 mcg), final dose (40 mcg) and post-stress. With either approach, four quad-screens are used for the four standard views. The images are then interpreted qualitatively, as described in Chapter 2.

4.2.3 *Hemodynamic Responses to Dobutamine Stress*

Dobutamine induces enhancement of left ventricular contractility at low doses, followed by increased systolic blood pressure, with heart-rates of over 100 beats/minute at doses >20 mcg/kg/minute. Cohen [12] has correlated the hemodynamic response with the presence and extent of coronary disease. Heart-rate was found to increase significantly, with peak heart-rates of about 120 beats/minute in most patients, reflecting a heart-rate increment of 40–50 beats/minute. Systolic blood pressure usually attains levels of about 170 mmHg in normotensive patients, due to an increment of 30 to 40 mmHg; Cohen found that only patients with 3–vessel disease failed to mount a significant blood pressure response. The rate-pressure product increases in all patients, with representative peak levels of 16,500–20,000 [11,12]. There is usually no significant change of diastolic blood pressure. As might be expected from the stepwise nature of the test, the development of ischemia occurs at lower dobutamine doses and at lower cardiac workloads in the presence of more extensive coronary disease. In our experience, however, there is too much overlap between groups for the hemodynamic response to be a reliable predictor of one-, two- or three-vessel coronary disease.

The physiologic responses to dobutamine may be tempered by beta-adrenoceptor blockade, which induces a state of competitive antagonism. Patients taking beta-blockers have been shown [11,13,14,20] to demonstrate a significantly lower peak heart-rate response (to a peak of 90 to 100 beats/minute), and a lower double-product (to levels of around 14,000), although the systolic blood pressure response is less attenuated. In a group of patients (almost all of whom were beta-blocked) who had no ischemia induced by a standard dobutamine protocol, atropine was shown to increase the heart-rate to 120 beats/minute, comparable to the levels attained in patients not taking beta-blocking agents [20].

Even in the presence of a maximal dobutamine stress, the hemodynamic responses to this agent are less than those usually recorded at maximal exercise stress. Four studies have reported on the physiologic responses to exercise and dobutamine stress, performed in the same patients [15,21–23]. In each study, although systolic blood pressure levels were comparable, the peak heart-rate and double product were significantly greater during exercise than dobutamine stress. Thus, while dobutamine is considered to be an "exercise simulating" drug, there are limitations to its correspondence with exercise stress. The effects of these disparities in the intensity of stress on the sensitivity of the test will be discussed further in a later section.

4.2.4 *Side-effects of Dobutamine Stress Testing*

The side-effects of dobutamine stress reflect the consequences of intense sympathomimetic stimulation. In our experience in 217 consecutive studies [17], 29% of patients developed significant dose-limiting side-effects, a frequency comparable with the 31% incidence reported by Salustri [13]. The end-points of dobutamine stress in our hands are summarized in Figure 4.2. About two-thirds of patients attained peak dose or achieved an ischemic end-point. Of the remaining patients, who stopped prematurely due to side-effects, the commonest problems were due to hypotension and arrhythmias. Other side-effects included: dyspnea, anxiety and vagal reactions, palpitations and formication, but these did not usually require test termination. Hypertension (we normally stop the test for systolic blood pressures >220/120) is surprisingly uncommon.

The frequency and severity of side-effects varies between studies; if all side-effects are included they may be recorded in up to 82% of patients [15], while a frequency of only 5% has been reported if only serious, dose-limiting side-effects are considered [11]. Some of this heterogeneity relates to the stress protocol employed; their incidence tends to be lower in studies where the test is terminated if patients achieve a target heart-rate or when echocardiographic evidence of ischemia is seen [11]. Similarly, side-effects were less prevalent in the series reported by Cohen [12], because patients with submaximal test responses were excluded.

Arrhythmias most commonly involve atrial and ventricular extrasystoles, non-sustained atrial and (less often) ventricular tachycardias, and rarely, atrial fibrillation and sustained ventricular tachycardia. In an experience of over 200 patients, we have not witnessed any sustained or life-threatening arrhythmias, a finding consistent with that reported from other centers, and contrary to previous concerns [24].

Hypotension (which is usually asymptomatic) has been variously defined, leading to some variability in its reported frequency. We terminate the test if the systolic blood pressure falls >20 mmHg; others have used a > 30 mmHg reduction [15] or a > 15 mmHg fall from baseline [11]. In our experience [17], hypotension is an unpredictable and frequent complication (occurring in 28%, although not necessarily provoking the termination of the test), unrelated to echocardiographic abnormalities or the presence or severity of coronary disease. This complication is usually due to the vasodilator effects of dobutamine, particularly if it appears suddenly after a dosage increment [25]. In some patients, it may reflect dynamic left ventricular outflow tract obstruction [26]. Data presented by Marcowitz [25] suggests that gradual falls in blood pressure are correlated to myocardial ischemia, and this may explain the attenuated blood pressure response in the group of patients with three-vessel disease reported by Cohen [13]. However, our experience is less consistent with hypotension being a marker of coronary disease – in 40 patients with sudden and 24 with gradual hypotension, the presence of coronary disease or ischemia in these groups did not differ from a control group of 164 patients without a hypotensive response.

As a consequence of these side-effects, dobutamine stress is contraindicated in patients with severe hypertension and serious arrhythmias. Nonetheless, while side-effects may concern the physician performing the test and compromise its sensitivity by limiting the maximum attained dose (see below), major complications are exceedingly rare and no deaths have been reported. One advantage of on-line echocardiographic imaging is that the extent and severity of ischemia may be better appreciated than they might with the electrocardiogram alone, or with pre- and post-stress imaging alone. This may permit termination of the stress before severe left ventricular dysfunction develops.

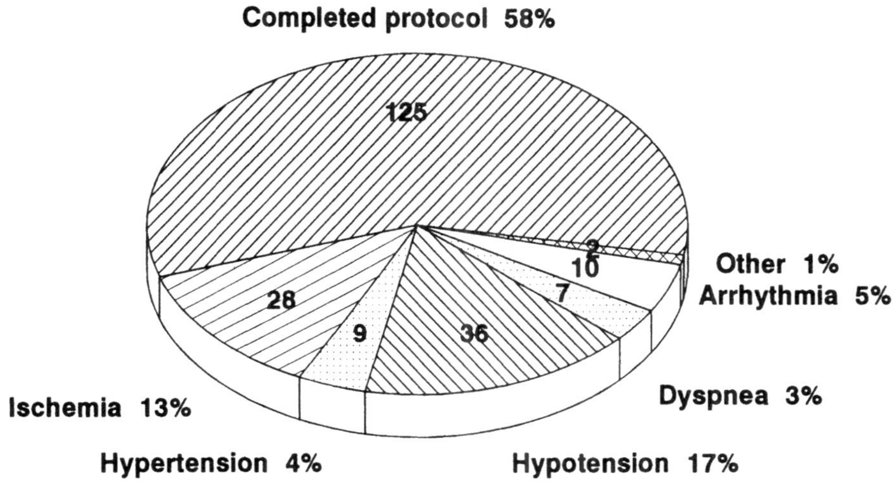

Figure 4.2. End-points of the dobutamine stress protocol in 217 unselected patients undergoing coronary angiography [17].

4.2.5 *Accuracy of Dobutamine Stress Testing*

In contrast to exercise testing [27], angina and electrocardiographic changes during dobutamine stress have limited accuracy except in patients with a high coronary disease probability. In those studies which permit a direct comparison of exercise and dobutamine data, the sensitivity of the former reproducibly exceeds that of the latter. These findings are discussed in more detail in Chapter 5, but to summarize our experience, we believe that dobutamine stress should necessarily be combined with an imaging technique.

The results of recent studies of dobutamine echocardiography are summarized in Table 4.1. The overall sensitivity for the detection of visually assessed stenoses of >50 or >70% varies from 68 to 95%. In comparison with quantitative angiography, dobutamine echocardiography has a sensitivity of 86% for the detection of stenoses with minimal lumenal diameters <1 mm [28]. These variations reflect differences in the study populations – our own experience has been interesting in this respect. Our initial experience with dobutamine echocardiography [29] comprised a trial where patients were carefully supervised, and were studied off therapy, under optimal conditions, yielding an overall sensitivity of 85%. As the clinical utility of the test became apparent, and routine clinical studies were incorporated into our experience, an increasing proportion of patients had a "suboptimal" test (either due to inability to complete the protocol or interference by beta-blocker therapy), and a lower sensitivity was reported [17].

As with exercise echocardiography, slightly higher sensitivities are reported for dobutamine echocardiography in patients with myocardial infarction, because the presence of a regional wall motion abnormality identifies

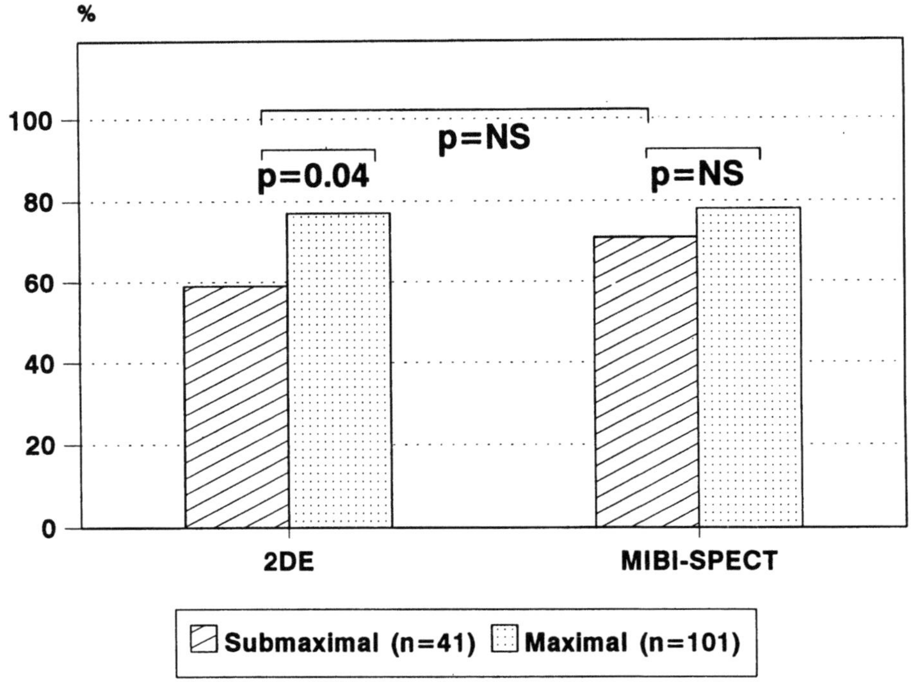

Figure 4.3. Relative effect of "submaximal" stress (failure to complete protocol or testing on beta-blocker therapy) on the sensitivity of dobutamine stress echocardiography (2DE) and perfusion scintigraphy (MIBI-SPECT) [17].

the presence of coronary disease, independent of the stress. The sensitivity of dobutamine echocardiography for the detection of single-vessel coronary disease is lower than for multivessel disease, and has been in the 40 to 70% range in most studies. Some heterogeneity in the accuracy of the test in this situation presumably reflects variations in the severity of single vessel coronary disease in different study groups.

The specificity of dobutamine echocardiography ranges from 82 to 100%. In our experience [17], no unifying feature accounts for these false positive results, which have a comparable frequency with those witnessed at exercise echocardiography.

Other sympathomimetic agents (epinephrine, isopreterenol) have been reported to have modest sensitivity in the diagnosis of coronary artery disease [30–32]. These agents have not achieved clinical acceptance because of safety concerns. Moreover, limitation of peak dose because of concerns regarding side-effects may restrict the attainable sensitivities.

4.2.6 *Evaluation of the Site and Extent of Coronary Disease Using Dobutamine Echocardiography*

The location, extent and severity of coronary disease are as readily studied using dobutamine as with exercise echocardiography. Using the standard assumptions about the distribution of coronary territories, Sawada reported the location of wall motion abnormality to correspond to the distribution of the stenosed vessel in 16 of 17 patients with single vessel disease [11]. The accuracy of dobutamine echocardiography for identification of coronary disease in the anterior and posterior circulations is equivalent [14,17].

The ability of exercise echocardiography to predict multivessel disease (Figure 4.4) is greater in those with than without previous myocardial infarction (see Chapter 3). The same is true of dobutamine stress; in 41 patients with a localized wall motion abnormality, Sawada found its sensitivity for remote disease (in the non-infarct-related artery) to be 81%, and its specificity to be 87% [11]. Similarly, studies of patients after myocardial infarction have shown a sensitivity of 85% and a specificity of 88% in the detection of multivessel disease [22]. Dobutamine echocardiography has therefore been proposed as an alternative to exercise testing for the detection of residual ischemia after myocardial infarction [21].

The recognition of multivessel disease in patients without previous infarction has been reported in up to 70% of patients with stenoses in >1 vessel [11]. This exceeds the levels reported for these patients using exercise echocardiography (see Chapter 3), and may reflect a greater propensity to continue the test once ischemia has occurred in one segment. Our experience has been less favorable; only 43% of patients with ≥2 vessel disease were recognised as such. This may reflect a tendency to focus on the most ischemic area (making other less ischemic regions appear normal), and may also occur if the pharmacologic study is terminated because of ischemia in one zone, before a second territory becomes ischemic.

In patients with multivessel disease, ischemia tends to have an earlier onset (Figure 4.5), at a lower dose of dobutamine and a lower heart-rate and rate-pressure product [11]. However, patients with severe single-vessel disease may also demonstrate an early onset of ischemia [14], so that while this relationship is a guide to lesion severity, we have not found the time or hemodynamic response at onset to be a useful predictor of multivessel disease.

In order to assess the ability of the test to appraise the extent of disease, free of assumptions about the distribution of individual coronary arteries, we compared the proportion of segments showing abnormal wall motion with an angiographic index of coronary disease extent (the Gensini score). This demonstrated a close correlation with an equivalent score of perfusion defect extent, although both underestimated the angiographic extent of disease as measured by the Gensini score [17].

Table 4.1. Sensitivity and specificity of dobutamine stress echocardiography.

Author	Reference	n	Peak dose mcg/kg/min	"Significant" CAD	Sensitivity – overall
Sawada	11	103	30	>50%	95% (n = 81)
Cohen	12	70	40	>70%	86% (n = 51)
Salustri	13	52	40	>50%	54% (n = 37)
Marcowitz	14	141	30	>50%	96% (n = 109)
Mazeika	15	50	20	>70%	78% (n = 36)
Previtali	16	35	40	>70%	68% (n = 28)
Marwick	17	217	40	>50%	72% (n = 142)

CAD = coronary artery disease, SVD = single vessel disease.

4.2.7 *Influence of Anti-anginal Therapy on the Results of Dobutamine Echocardiography*

As the development of ischemia is a sine que non of developing abnormal regional function, anti-ischemic therapy may be expected to reduce the sensitivity of stress echocardiography. Thus, beta-blockers, calcium antagonists and combined therapy have been shown to reduce the sensitivity of dipyridamole stress echocardiography. Surprisingly, the influence of anti-anginal therapy on the sensitivity of dobutamine echocardiography has been a matter of some dispute, with several series failing to document an effect [11,13,14]. These results may clouded by a degree of selection bias, as patients with more symptomatic coronary disease (which is therefore more severe and more likely to precipitate ischemia) are more likely to be on treatment. In our experience, false negatives have correlated with patients who failed to complete the protocol due to the development of side-effects and/or who took beta adrenoreceptor antagonists on the day of the test; these situations may be an indication for combining the test with perfusion scintigraphy, which is not so severely compromised by these features (Figure 4.3). In the experience of McNeill [20], patients on beta-blockers accounted for 94% of patients who failed to attain >85% of age-predicted maximal heart-rate, and had a negative test result. In this situation, the administration of atropine (up to 1 mg), after the conclusion of the dobutamine protocol has been shown to intensify the hemodynamic response to dobutamine, and may enhance the sensitivity of dobutamine stress testing, without reducing specificity or inducing serious side-effects.

4.2.8 *Should Dobutamine Echocardiography Be Considered in Patients Who Are Able to Exercise?*

The above sections have focussed on the use of non-exercise stress in those patients who are unable to exercise. Even in patients who are able to exercise,

Sensitivity – SVD	Specificity CAD	Sensitivity normal RWM	Specificity normal RWM
89% (n = 38)	77% (n = 22)	89% (n = 35)	85% (n = 20)
69% (n = 16)	95% (n = 19)	–	–
40% (n = 20)	80% (n = 15)	63% (n = 24)	80% (n = 15)
95% (n = 62)	66% (n = 32)	87% (n = 30)	91% (n = 23)
50% (n = 12)	93% (n = 14)	70% (n = 23)	100% (n = 13)
50% (n = 16)	100% (n = 7)	–	–
66% (n = 68)	83% (n = 75)	–	–

pharmacologic approaches are attractive. The technical demands of acquiring good images in an exercising, tachypneic patient are substantial, and although ameliorated by post-stress imaging, this is at the cost of a reduction of sensitivity. Pharmacologic stress has the attraction of offering imaging at peak stress, without the difficulty of performing the study in an exercising patient. Apart from the practical aspects, the ability to readily examine the time of onset of ischemia is not available with pre- and post-treadmill imaging, and less feasible during bicycle stress than during pharmacologic protocols. Exercise techniques are more dependent on the interpretation of digitized cine-loop images, with the inherent problems of sampling error due to non-representative beats or views.

Echocardiographic responses to stress have been compared between dobutamine and exercise in three studies [23,33,34]. Using supine bicycle exercise in patients off medical therapy, Cohen [33] reported a sensitivity of 76% for exercise, and 86% for dobutamine stress – this difference being non-significant, for both patients with single- and multi-vessel disease. The specificity of both tests was 87%. In 48 patients with suspected coronary disease and with studies of good quality, Hoffman [34] reported supine bicycle echocardiography to have a feasibility of 88%, a sensitivity of 84%, and a specificity of 88%. The respective figures for dobutamine were 90%, 88% and 84%. However, although bicycle and dobutamine echocardiography produced analogous results in these studies, both involved supine bicycle stress and excluded patients with suboptimal studies. Preliminary comparisons of arbutamine with exercise have also been reported, showing similar levels of accuracy [9]. However, both dobutamine and arbutamine induce a lower workload on the heart than exercise. The implications of this under routine clinical circumstances need to be addressed for both compounds.

In our comparison of dobutamine and exercise echocardiography, we attempted to reproduce the circumstances of routine clinical practice [23]. In this study, the overall accuracy of dobutamine echocardiography (64%) was less than that of bicycle exercise stress (85%, $p < 0.0001$) in 86 unselected

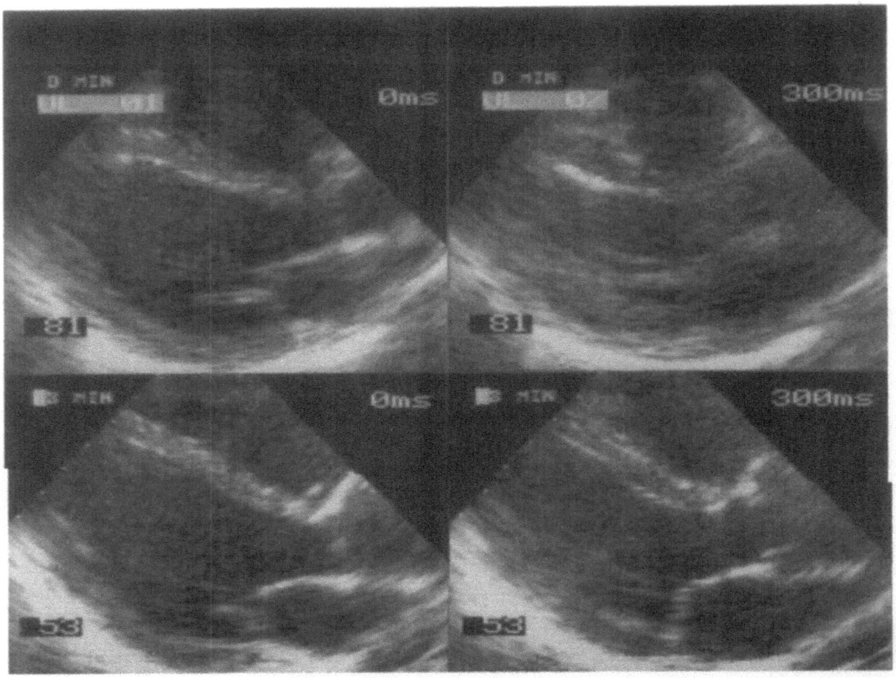

Figure 4.4. Freeze-frame and traced diastolic (left) and systolic (right) images before and after low-dose (5 mcg/kg/minute) dobutamine. The anteroseptal and posterior walls show reduced excursion and thickening (arrows), and the systolic cavity size has increased. The multiple

patients without myocardial infarction. While the specificity of dobutamine echocardiography (83%) was somewhat greater than that at peak exercise (80%), the relative sensitivities were dependent upon the presence of anti-anginal treatment and the ability of patients to complete the dobutamine protocol. In patients not taking beta-blockers on the day of the test and able to complete the dobutamine protocol ("optimal" test, n = 22) the sensitivity of dobutamine echocardiography (73%) was not significantly different from that of exercise echocardiography (87%). In contrast, in those with a suboptimal dobutamine stress test, the sensitivity (41%) was less than that obtainable with exercise (94%, $p < 0.0001$). These data were supported by the development of ST segment depression, which occurred with comparable frequency during dobutamine and exercise stress in the "optimal" group (59% vs 77%) but was less frequent during dobutamine than exercise in the suboptimal dose group (15% vs 73%, $p < 0.01$). The effect of submaximal dobutamine stress had less impact on the overall sensitivity of dobutamine stress perfusion scintigraphy (65%), which was not significantly different from that of exercise scintigraphy (73%). The difference in the sensitivity between dobutamine and exercise stress echocardiography parallels the greater cardiac workload

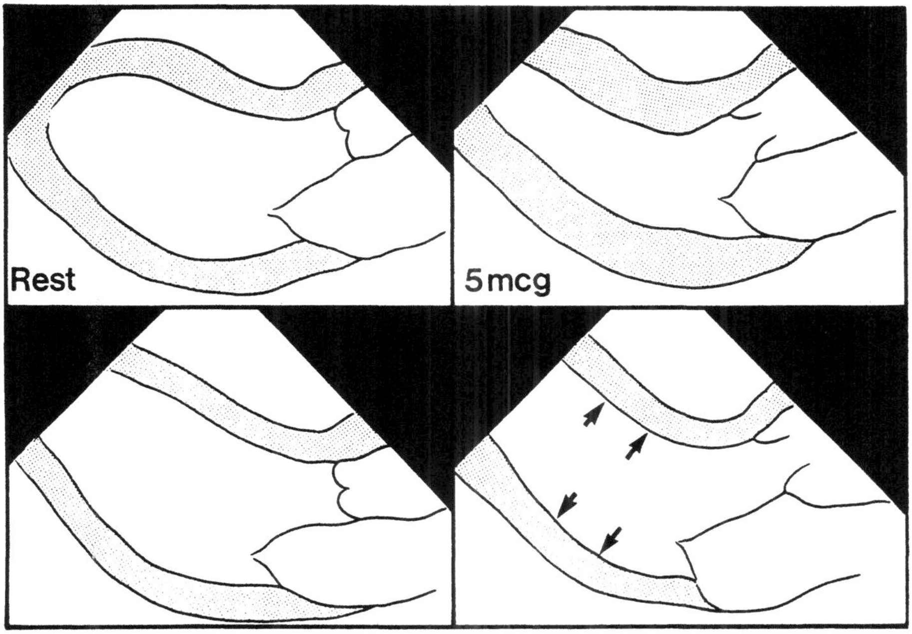

involved segments and early onset of ischemia concur with the finding of multivessel coronary artery disease at angiography.

imposed by exercise (Figure 4.6). Thus, the sensitivity and accuracy of dobutamine echocardiography are only comparable to those of exercise echocardiography in patients able to undergo an optimal dobutamine test.

Moreover, in our experience [23], exercise induced more ischemia than dobutamine, even when the comparison was restricted to the 28 patients with coronary disease who demonstrated stress-induced wall motion abnormalities at both tests. At echocardiography, the extent of wall motion abnormality at exercise (34 ± 18% of left ventricular segments) exceeded the extent demonstrated as ischemic using dobutamine stress (15 ± 8%, $p < 0.0001$). Similarly, the extent of perfusion defects at exercise (29 ± 12% of left ventricular segments) exceeded the extent of defects using dobutamine stress (22 ± 11%, $p = 0.02$), in the 33 patients with coronary disease who showed stress-induced perfusion defects at both tests.

We also examined the relative feasibility of dobutamine and exercise stress, using a qualitative, four point scale of image quality (described in Chapter 2) and a similar three point scale of diagnostic confidence. Dobutamine echocardiograms provided higher quality images than those attainable using the bicycle. Of the 86 dobutamine echocardiograms, 20 were of A quality, 53 of B quality, 11 of C quality and 2 of D quality, compared with

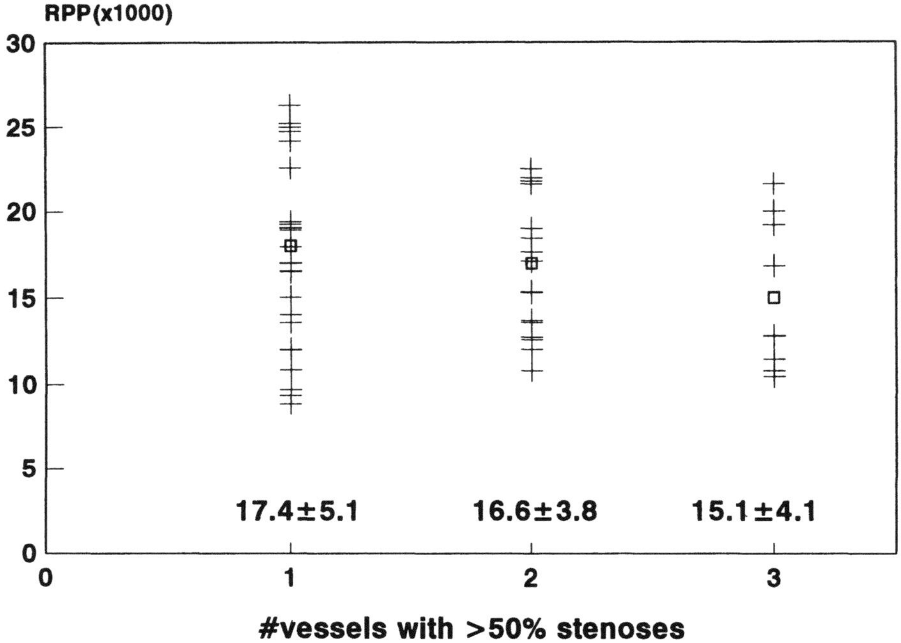

Figure 4.5. Rate-pressure product at the onset of ischemia in 46 patients with 1, 2 and 3 vessel disease and a positive dobutamine stress echocardiogram. There is a trend towards the onset of ischemia at lower rate-pressure product with increasing severity of coronary disease.

3, 46, 29, and 8 studies of these respective qualities with exercise. Thus, 73 dobutamine echocardiograms were of excellent or good quality (85%), compared with 49 at exercise (57%, $p < 0.001$). The opposite relationship applied to diagnostic certainty, which was greatest with exercise echocardiography; 15 of the 86 dobutamine echocardiograms (17%) were interpreted with a high level of confidence, compared with 32 exercise studies (37%, $p = 0.004$). Moderate diagnostic confidence was attained in 47 dobutamine and 31 exercise echocardiograms, and low levels of diagnostic certainty were present in 24 dobutamine and 23 bicycle studies.

In summary, the technical facility of dobutamine echocardiography permits the acquisition of better quality images than are available with exercise. However, this benefit is outweighed by the fact that dobutamine imposes a lower workload on the heart, with the consequence of smaller, less severely ischemic foci, which are more difficult to recognise. Finally, dobutamine appears to be a less robust stress than exercise, and its sensitivity is significantly compromised by submaximal stress.

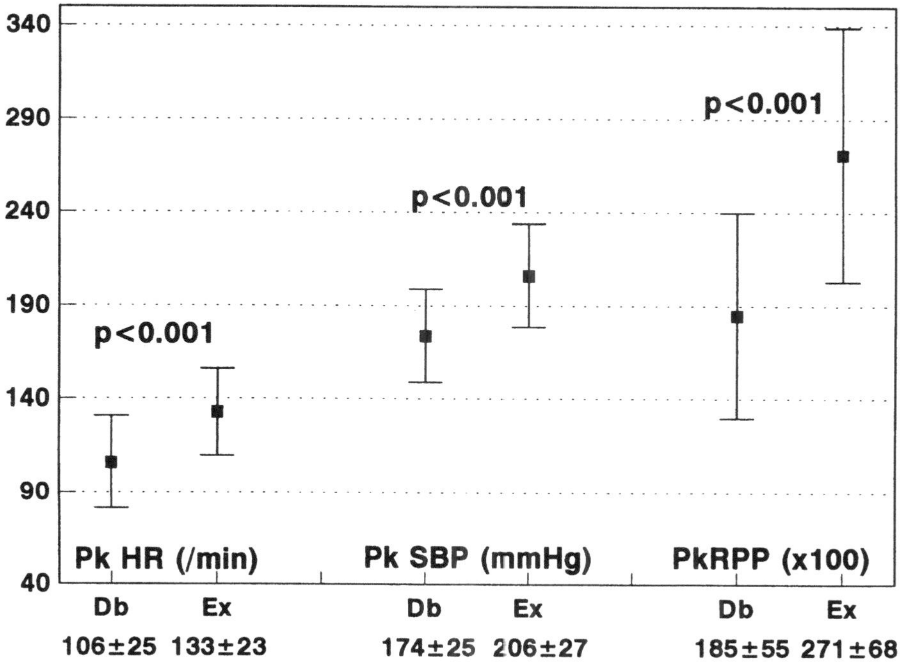

Figure 4.6. Heart-rate (HR), systolic blood pressure (SBP) and rate-pressure product (RPP) responses at peak effect (Pk) during dobutamine and exercise stress in 86 patients with suspected coronary disease.

4.3 Exercise Simulation Using Pacing Stress

While pharmacologic stress echocardiography has been found to be accurate, these tests are contraindicated in some patients, and side-effects may limit their feasibility in others. Atrial pacing stress, although more invasive, has the advantage of avoiding these sequellae.

Pacing induces myocardial ischemia [35,36] by increasing myocardial oxygen consumption (due to increased heart-rate), and reducing subendocardial perfusion [37]. This technique has unique advantages, including the ability to immediately terminate the stress if the patient develops complications, and the capacity to achieve a pre-determined heart-rate in almost all patients. The use of pacing for stress testing has involved atrial stimulation, either transvenously or via the esophagus, as ventricular pacing itself causes both abnormal regional contractility and abnormal perfusion. Of these, only the transesophageal route has gained acceptance as a routine stress modality.

Transesophageal atrial pacing (TAP) using a "pill electrode" has been combined with transthoracic imaging for nearly 10 years [38]. A typical protocol takes about 11 minutes, starting at a heart-rate of 110 beats per minute, increasing in 2 minute intervals to a rate of 150 per minute. Atropine

Table 4.2. Sensitivity and specificity of atrial-pacing stress echocardiography.

Author	Reference	n	Methodology	Feasibility	Sensitivity – overall	Sensitivity – SVD
Lambertz	41	50	TAP-TEE	100%	93% (n = 46)	85% (n = 20)
Kamp	42	71	TAP-TEE	99%	83% (n = 52)	69% (n = 13)
Zabalgoitia	43	36	TAP-TEE	90%*	90% (n = 21)	100% (n = 14)

* Feasibility in complete unselected series of 86 patients.

may be required to overcome Wenckebach atrioventricular block, which may become apparent at high pacing rates. The test is performed using the normal precautions for stress testing, with ECG and echocardiographic monitoring. The usual endpoints are the completion of the pacing protocol, or the development of extensive ischemia as defined by severe chest pain, severe ECG changes or extensive wall motion abnormalities. Very favorable results have been obtained by the use of atrial pacing in combination with echocardiography (Table 4.2). In a large series, the sensitivity of this test was shown to be 89%, with a specificity of 84% [39].

The ability to cease pacing and suddenly return to a low (though not necessarily resting) heart-rate may be of particular value in Doppler stress testing, as the hemodynamic sequellae of ischemia take some time to resolve, even after the ischemic stimulus dissipates. Studies using this methodology have shown a pattern consistent with reduced ventricular compliance, with reduction of rapid filling and enhancement of active filling [40]. These changes are difficult to discern with other forms of stress, because the active and passive filling waves tend to merge during tachycardias. Similarly, the same maneuver may assist in the combination of stress testing with color-flow Doppler as the use of low frame-rates may pose a problem at high heart-rates. Despite these advantages, however, this technique has not become widely used because in the experience of many centers, esophageal pacing may be poorly tolerated.

A newer development has been the use of TAP in combination with transesophageal echocardiography (TEE). The attachment of the pacing electrodes to the TEE probe enhances their contact with the esophagus, reducing stimulation energy (because smaller currents are required to attain atrial capture), and enhancing patient tolerance. The technique of TAP-TEE involves placement of the TEE probe in the usual fashion. The electrodes are attached 7 to 12 cm proximal to the tip, so that when the transducer is in the stomach, they are positioned directly adjacent to the left atrium.

Specificity	Pacing ECG – sensitivity	Exercise ECG – sensitivity	Pacing ECG – specificity	Exercise ECG – specificity
100% (n = 9)	49% (n = 46)	53% (n = 46)	67% (n = 9)	50% (n = 9)
94% (n = 18)	52% (n = 40)	50% (n = 48)	82% (n = 17)	83% (n = 18)
93% (n = 14)	43% (n = 14)	–	100% (n = 11)	–

Pacing is usually started at 110 beats/minute and increased in 10 beat/minute increments every 2 minutes until a rate of 150/minute, which is maintained for 5 minutes. The test is performed using the normal precautions and endpoints for stress testing, with ECG and TEE monitoring. In the three reported studies to date [41–43], the sensitivity and specificity of this approach have been in the range of 90% (Table 4.2). These very favorable findings have been paralleled by similar findings using transesophageal echocardiography and dipyridamole stress [44], implying that the accuracy of the technique pertains more to high-quality imaging than the chosen stress modality. The approach is not without problems, however. In relation to TAP, the need to stimulate the esophagus has prevented esophageal views from being acquired – thus all imaging has been performed in the transgastric plane (being limited to the short axis view when using a single-plane probe). This may be ameliorated by multiple electrodes higher on the probe (to permit longitudinal transgastric views), or with use of the multiplane probe. Second, the insertion of the transesophageal probe in an awake patient may itself provoke hemodynamic changes and hence ischemia, so that "resting" TEE images may not be truly acquired at rest. Third, the equipment requirement is greater than that needed for the alternative approaches. Finally, given the invasive nature of this test, it seems unlikely that stress TEE will become the stress echocardiographic modality of first choice for all patients, although it is clearly of benefit in those with suboptimal transthoracic images, patients intolerant to pharmacologic stresses, or those in whom pacing rather than pharmacologic stress is attractive for safety reasons.

A study comparing TAP and exercise echocardiography has shown similar levels of accuracy [45]. The former was shown to be more feasible (in 95%), although the lower feasibility of exercise echocardiography in that study (80%) reflects a success rate somewhat lower than the usually obtained levels (see Chapter 3).

4.6 Conclusion

Currently available data suggest that pacing and dobutamine stress (provided that the dobutamine protocol is completed) are able to provide similar levels of accuracy to exercise echocardiography. As pacing is unpleasant, we limit the use of this stress to patients with contra-indications to dobutamine infusion. Atropine may be a useful adjunct to any stressor if a higher heart-rate response is desired. In patients with a poor transthoracic window, transesophageal echocardiography should be considered, with pacing or pharmacologic stressors.

The performance of non-exercise stress echocardiography is more feasible than with exercise, and the training requirement for the acquisition of exercise images is probably greater than for echocardiography during pharmacologic stress or pacing stress. On the other hand, a number of considerations favor the use of exercise stress in those who can perform it. Exercise stress provides useful ECG data (which are less accurate with pharmacologic stressors), yields important data regarding functional capacity and prognosis, and gives results which are readily extrapolated to everyday life. Based on these considerations, exercise echocardiography, if practicable and in expert hands, currently appears to offer more data than the non-exercise approaches. Our current practice is to limit the use of exercise simulating techniques to patients who are unable to perform maximal exercise.

References

1. Baudhuin T, Marwick T, D'Hondt AM, Melin JA, Detry JM. Diagnosis of coronary artery disease in elderly patients: Safety and efficacy of dobutamine echocardiography. Eur Heart J 1993;14:799–803.
2. Josephson MA, Brown BG, Hecht HS *et al.* Noninvasive detection and localization of coronary stenoses in patients: Comparison of resting dipyridamole and exercise thallium-201 myocardial perfusion imaging. Am Heart J 1982;103:1008–13.
3. Vasu MA, O'Keefe DD, Kapellakis GZ *et al.* Myocardial oxygen consumption: Effects of epinephrine, isoproterenol, dopamine, norepinephrine and dobutamine. Am J Physiol 1978;235:H237–H241.
4. Warltier DC, Zyvoloski M, Gross GJ, Hardman HF, Brooks HL. Redistribution of myocardial blood flow distal to a dynamic coronary arterial stenosis by sympathomimetic amines: Comparison of dopamine, dobutamine and isoproterenol. Am J Cardiol 1981;48:269–79.
5. Vatner SF, Baig H. Importance of heart rate in determining the effects of sympathomimetic amines on regional myocardial function and blood flow in conscious dogs with acute myocardial ischemia. Circ Res 1979;45:793–803.
6. Fujita T, Ajisaka R, Matsumoto R *et al.* Isoproterenol infusion stress two-dimensional echocardiography in diagnosis of coronary artery disease in elderly patients: Comparison with the other stress testing methods. Jpn Heart J 1986;27:287–97.
7. Tuttle RR, Mills J. Dobutamine: development of a new catecholamine to selectively increase cardiac contractility. Circ Res 1975;36:185–96.
8. McGillem MJ, DeBoe SF, Friedman HZ, Mancini GBJ. The effects of dopamine and

dobutamine on regional function in the presence of rigid coronary stenoses and subcritical impairments of reactive hyperemia. Am Heart J 1988;115:970–7.

9. Ginzton LE, Appleton C, Mohuiddin S *et al.* Arbutamine, a new agent for diagnosing coronary artery disease: Comparison with exercise testing. J Am Coll Cardiol 1993;21:229A.
10. Ruffolo RR Jr, Spradlin TA, Pollock GD, Waddell JE, Murphy PJ. Alpha and beta effects of the streoisomers of dobutamine. J Pharmacol Exp Ther 1981;219:447–52.
11. Sawada SG, Segar DS, Ryan T *et al.* Echocardiographic detection of coronary artery disease during dobutamine infusion. Circulation 1991;83:1605–14.
12. Cohen JL, Greene TO, Ottenweller J, Binenbaum SZ, Wilchfort SD, Kim CS. Dobutamine digital echocardiography for detecting coronary artery disease. Am J Cardiol 1991;67:1311–8.
13. Salustri A, Fioretti PR, Pozzoli MMA, McNeill AJ, Roelandt JR. Dobutamine stress echocardiography: its role in the diagnosis of coronary artery disease. Eur Heart J 1992;13:70–7.
14. Marcowitz P, Armstrong WF. Accuracy of dobutamine stress echocardiography in detecting coronary artery disease. Am J Cardiol 1992;69:1269–73.
15. Mazieka PK, Nadazdin A, Oakley CM. Dobutamine stress echocardiography fpr detection and assessment of coronary artery disease. J Am Coll Cardiol 1992;19:1203–11.
16. Previtali M, Lanzarini L, Ferrario M, Tortorici M, Mussini A, Montemartini C. Dobutamine versus dipyridamole echocardiography in coronary artery disease. Circulation 1991;83(Suppl III):27–31.
17. Marwick T, D'Hondt A, Baudhuin T *et al.* Optimal use of dobutamine stress for the detection and evaluation of coronary artery disease: Combination with echocardiography, scintigraphy or both? J Am Coll Cardiol 1993;22:159–67.
18. Pennell DJ, Underwood SR, Swanton RH, Walker JM, Ell PJ. Dobutamine thallium myocardial perfusion tomography. J Am Coll Cardiol 1991;18:1471–9.
19. Mason JR, Palac RT, Freeman ML *et al.* Thallium scintigraphy during dobutamine infusion: Nonexercise-dependent screening test for coronary disease. Am Heart J 1984;107:481–5.
20. McNeil AJ, Fioretti PM, El-Said EM, Salustri A, de Feyter PJ, Roelandt JR. Enhanced sensitivity for detection of coronary artery disease by addition of atropine to dobutamine stress echocardiography. Am J Cardiol 1992;70:41–6.
21. Mannering D, Cripps, T, Leech G *et al.* The dobutamine stress test as an alternative to exercise testing after acute myocardial infarction. Br Heart J 1988;59:521–6.
22. Berthe C, Pierard LA, Hiernaux M *et al.* Predicting the extent and location of coronary artery disease in acute myocardial infarction by echocardiography during dobutamine infusion. Am J Cardiol 1986;58:1167–72.
23. Marwick T, D'Hondt A-M, Mairesse G *et al.* Should patients able to exercise undergo exercise or dobutamine echocardiography? (abstract) Eur Heart J 1993;14:454.
24. Furiasse JG, Labarre TR, Moran JF, Henkin RE, Scanlon PJ. Malignant ventricular arrhythmias during dobutamine thallium stress testing [abstract]. Circulation 1985;72(Suppl III):424.
25. Marcowitz PA, Bach DS, Markarian M, Mathias WS, Armstrong WF. Implications of a hypotensive response during dobutamine stress echocardiography [abstract]. J Am Coll Cardiol 1992;19:360A.
26. Mazieka PK, Nadazdin A, Oakley CM. Clinical significance of abrupt vasodepression during dobutamine stress echocardiography. Am J Cardiol 1992;69:1484–7.
27. Gianrossi R, Detrano R, Mulvihill D *et al.* Exercise-induced ST depression in the diagnosis of coronary artery disease: A meta-analysis. Circulation 1989;80:87–98.
28. Segar DS, Brown SE, Sawada SG, Ryan T, Feigenbaum H. Dobutamine stress echocardiography: Correlation with coronary lesion severity as determined by quantitative angiography. J Am Coll Cardiol 1992;19:1197–202.
29. Marwick T, Willemart B, D'Hondt AM *et al.* Selection of the Optimal Non-Exercise Stress for the Evaluation of Ischemic Regional Myocardial Dysfunction and Malperfusion:

Comparison of Dobutamine and Adenosine using Echocardiography and Tc-99 m MIBI Single Photon Emission Computed Tomography. Circulation 1993;87:345–54.
30. Bernstein RF, Gross RG, Child JS, Krivokapich J, Thessonboom S. Isopreterenol stress echocardiography: A new method for detecting coronary artery disease [abstract]. Circulation 1984;70(Suppl II):184.
31. Ferrara N, Leosco D, Longobardi G *et al.* Use of the epinephrine test in diagnosis of coronary artery disease. Am J Cardiol 1986;58:256–60.
32. Wisenberg G, Zawadowski AG, Gebhardt VA *et al.* Dopamine: Its potential for inducing ischemic left ventricular dysfunction. J Am Coll Cardiol 1985;6:84–92.
33. Cohen JL, Duvvuri S, George A *et al.* Dobutamine versus exercise digital echocardiography for detecting coronary artery disease[abstract]. J Am Coll Cardiol 1992;19:32A.
34. Hoffmann R, Lethen H, Kleinhans E, Flachskampf FA, Hanrath P. Comparison of bicycle and dobutamine stress echocardiography for identification of coronary artery disease [abstract]. Circulation 1991;84:II–476.
35. Pasternac A, Gorlin R, Sonnenblick EH, Haft HI, Kemp HG. Abnormalities of ventricular motion induced by atrial pacing in coronary artery disease. Circulation 1972;45:1195–205.
36. Heller GV, Aroesty JM, Parker JA *et al.* The pacing stress test: thallium-201 myocardial imaging after atrial pacing. Diagnostic value in detecting coronary artery disease compared with exercise testing. J Am Coll Cardiol 1984;3:1197–204.
37. Becker L. Effect of tachycardia on left ventricular blood flow distribution during coronary occlusion. Am J Physiol 1976;230:1072–7.
38. Iliceto S, Sorino M, D'Ambrosio G *et al.* Detection of coronary artery disease by two-dimensional echocardiography and transesophageal atrial pacing. J Am Coll Cardiol 1985;5:1188–97.
39. Iliceto S, Sorino M, D'Ambrosio G *et al.* Atrial pacing in the detection and evaluation of coronary artery disease. Eur Heart J 1986;7(Suppl C):59–67.
40. Iliceto S, Amico A, Marangelli V, D'Ambrosio G, Rizzon P. Doppler echocardiographic evaluation of the effect of atrial pacing-induced ischemia on left ventricular filling in patients with coronary artery disease. J Am Coll Cardiol 1988;11:953–61.
41. Lambertz H, Kreis A, Trumper H, Hanrath P. Simultaneous transesophageal atrial pacing and transesophageal echocardiography: A new method of stress echocardiography. J Am Coll Cardiol 1990;16:1143–53.
42. Kamp O, De Cock CC, Funke Kupper AJ, Roos JP, Visser CA. Simultaneous transesophageal two-dimensional echocardiography and atrial pacing for detecting coronary artery disease. Am J Cardiol 1992;69:1412–6.
43. Zabalgoitia M, Gandhi DK, Abi-Mansour P, Yarnold PR, Moushmoush B, Rosenblum J. Transesophageal stress echocardiography: Detection of coronary disease in patients with normal left ventricular contractility. Am Heart J 1991;122:1456–63.
44. Agati L, Renzi M, Sciomer S *et al.* Transesophageal dipyridamole echocardiography for diagnosis of coronary artery disease. J Am Coll Cardiol 1992;19:765–70.
45. Iliceto S, Sorino M, D'Ambrosio G *et al.* Comparison of post-exercise and transesophageal atrial pacing two-dimensional echocardiography for detection of coronary artery disease. Am J Cardiol 1986;57:547–5.

5 Stress Echocardiography with Vasoactive Agents

Exercise and dobutamine stress induce ischemia by increasing myocardial oxygen requirements to a level which exceeds the ability of a stenosed coronary artery to satisfy the increased demand (see Chapters 3 and 4) Ischemia in most ambulatory situations is caused by oxygen demand out stripping supply, but it may be combined with reduction in coronary supply due to vasospasm or coronary steal This "supply-side" ischemia may be replicated during stress testing, either using dipyridamole as a convenient form of pharmacologic stress, or using ergotamine to specifically investigate the presence of a vasoactive mechanism of ischemia

5.1 Vasodilator Stressors

5 1 1 *Mechanism of Action*

As in the case of the exercise simulating drugs, more than one vasodilator stress agent (dipyridamole and adenosine) is available In contrast to the differing profiles of the sympathomimetic agents, however, the vasodilators differ more subtly Dipyridamole exerts its effects indirectly, through increasing endogenous adenosine levels, by reduction of cellular re-uptake and metabolism [1,2] Variability of its effects on these processes may account for "dipyridamole insensitivity" [3] Adenosine is a powerful vasodilator of a strength equivalent to that of papaverine [4] Thus, despite their final common pathway, dipyridamole and adenosine differ in their time of onset (respectively 4 to 8 minutes and immmediate), their duration of effect (respective half lives being 6 hours and 10 seconds), and in the intensity of their side-effects (which are more intense, and more transient, with adenosine) Dipyridamole has the benefit of a longer clinical experience as a stress agent [5]

Based upon studies demonstrating increased coronary flow without increased oxygen requirements [6], dipyridamole was initially used as an anti anginal agent However, before long, it was found to precipitate ischemia [7], and the mechanism of this was reported to be coronary "steal" – a phenomenon whereby blood which supplies compromised tissue is "stolen" by well perfused regions after administration of the drug While dipyridamole

T.H Marwick, Stress Echocardiography 81–94.

was subsequently reported – predominantly in the German literature [8] – as a non-exercise provocative agent for the stress ECG, it has gained most attention in the dipyridamole thallium protocol [9]. Its mechanism of action in this context is readily understandable, as the drug induces maximal coronary vasodilation throughout the heart, leading to flow heterogeneity in the presence of significant coronary stenoses and therefore apparent perfusion defects, with or without ischemia being provoked in a functional or metabolic sense.

The diagnosis of coronary disease at stress echocardiography mandates the induction of regional wall motion abnormalities (and hence ischemia), and several means have been proposed for the provocation of ischemia with dipyridamole [8,10,11]. Coronary steal is believed to be the main mechanism – this may be "vertical" or "horizontal" through the left ventricular wall. Vertical steal (subepicardial from subendocardial) occurs because of the depressurization of the microcirculation in response to vasodilation, causing vessels to collapse under the greater extravascular pressure of the subendocardium. Horizontal steal (non-stenosed from stenosed territory) is caused by reduced flow to collaterals from normal vessels after the runoff from these increases in response to vasodilation. Non-steal mechanisms may involve the effects of dipyridamole upon the stenosis, perfusion pressure, and even demand-induced ischemia. Profound vasodilation of the microcirculation may provoke "collapse" of the stenosis due to a reduction of lateral pressure induced by increased flow. Systemic vasodilation may compound these mechanisms by reduction of diastolic coronary perfusion pressure. Ischemia may be perpetuated by increased cardiac workload due to increased sympathetic activity secondary to angina, and coronary spasm may also play a minor role. However, despite all of these putative mechanisms, myocardial metabolic studies using positron emission tomography have suggested that metabolic evidence of ischemia is uncommon even in patients showing flow heterogeneity in response to dipyridamole [12].

5.1.2 *Vasodilator Stress Protocols*

Coffee, tea and cola drinks should be avoided for 12 hours before the examination, as xanthines antagonise the effects of dipyridamole on adenosine metabolism [13], as well as by direct competitive inhibition of adenosine activity. Patients are also usually advised to fast for a few hours before the test, as dipyridamole may induce nausea.

The procedure should be undertaken in the stress laboratory, or a similarly equipped room.In addition to the usual resuscitation equipment, aminophylline and intravenous nitrates should be available for the treatment of occasional, severe ischemia. The patient is prepared for stress testing in the usual fashion, and an intravenous line is inserted. For dipyridamole stress, we attempt to use a large proximal arm vein, as this compound is strongly alkaline and tends to cause local discomfort if not well diluted by venous

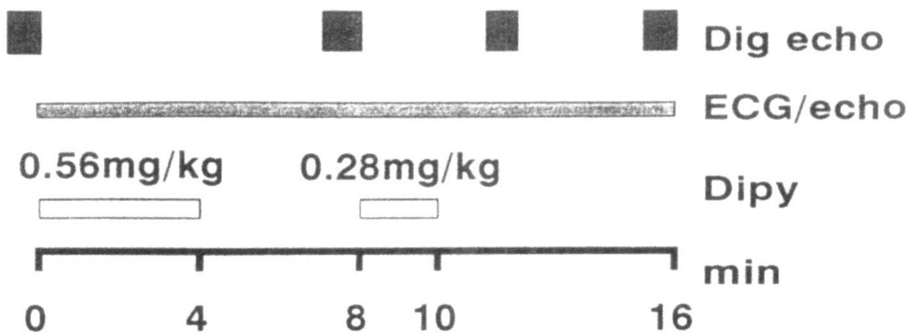

Figure 5.1. High-dose dipyridamole echocardiography protocol, illustrating two-stage infusion under echocardiographic (echo) and ECG monitoring, with digitization (dig) at rest, before and twice following the second dose.

blood. The most commonly administered dose for intravenous dipyridamole for myocardial perfusion imaging is 0.14 mg/kg/min [14]; oral dipyridamole has been used for echocardiography [15], but is not recommended now that the parenteral form is readily available, as its absorbtion and time-course of effects are erratic. The usual 4 minute infusion protocol for myocardial perfusion scintigraphy [0.56 mg/kg) has been found to produce unsatisfactory levels of sensitivity for stress echocardiography (Figure 5.1), but may be significantly enhanced by an additional 2 minutes of infusion if the initial response is negative and no major side-effects have appeared [16]. Electrocardiographic and echocardiographic monitoring is continued throughout the study and recorded on video-tape. Digitized images are saved at rest, before the start of the second dose (8 minutes), after the second dose (12 minutes, which is the commonest time for the onset of ischemia), and at 16 minutes. As positivity after 18 minutes is extremely rare, some authorities routinely administer 50 to 75 mg of aminophylline, to counteract the effects of dipyridamole, and to induce coronary spasm (in case ischemia is in part caused by this process). We recommend an individualized approach to the use of this antidote, depending on the presence and extent of ischemia induced, the overall left ventricular function, and the clinical state of the patient. Larger doses of aminophylline (200 mg or more) may be needed to reverse severe ischemia.

Adenosine is a direct-acting drug, which rapidly achieves steady state, and with biological effects of rapid onset [4]. It is therefore suitable for injection using an incremental dose schedule. Early studies using the drug in combination with myocardial perfusion scintigraphy [17,18], started at low doses. The original echocardiographic study with this agent employed a peak dose of 0.14 mg/kg/min [19]. We have used increments of 0.10, 0.14 and 0.18 mg/kg/min, in 3 minute stages [20], which duplicates the "high-dose" dipyridamole protocol, as long as the peak dose is tolerated. Digitized images

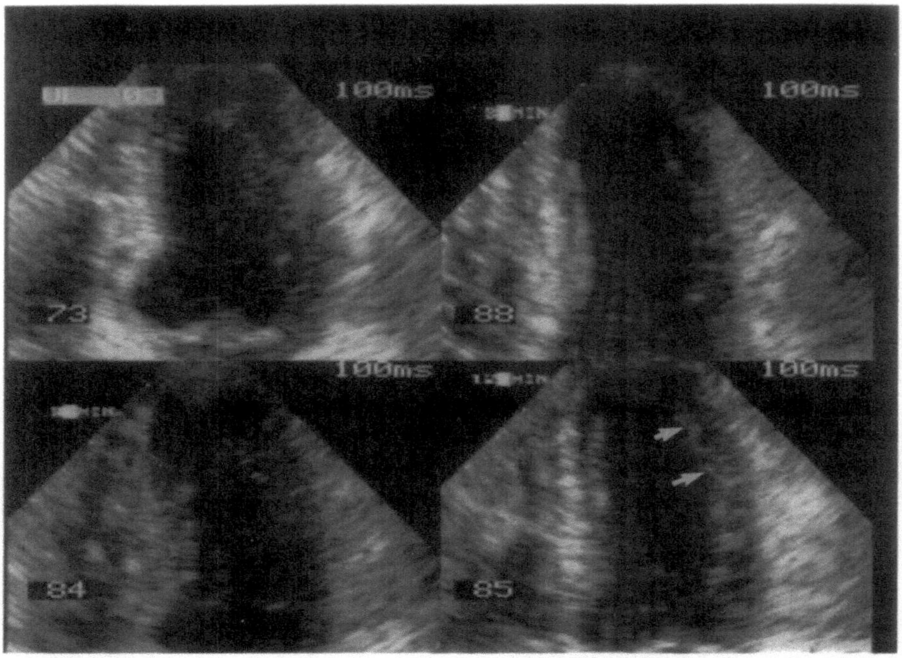

Figure 5.2. Freeze-frame systolic images at rest (upper left), before (upper right) and after (lower frames) the second dose of a high-dose dipyridamole echocardiography protocol. The anterior wall demonstrates reduced excursion after the second dose (arrows). Note the absence of a hyperkinetic response to stress (contrast with Figure 4.1), and a minor increment of heart-rate.

are acquired at the end of each 3 minute interval. Aminophylline is not required, as effects resolve within a minute of stopping the infusion.

Studies are interpreted by comparison of resting and stress images, using a similar approach to that employed for exercise and dobutamine. However, because of the lack of a major inotropic component to vasodilator stress (Figure 5.2), the development of hyperkinesis is not considered, and deterioration of hypokinetic segments is more readily ascribed to ischemia (as wall stress is not significantly altered). Thus, ischemia at vasodilator echocardiography is identified by the presence of a new or worsening wall motion abnormality.

5.1.3 *Hemodynamic Effects of Vasodilator Stress Agents*

Unlike exercise and dobutamine stresses, dipyridamole exerts only minor effects on cardiac workload. Irrespective of the presence or absence of coronary artery disease [21], patients undergoing a high-dose protocol show a significant increment of heart-rate (to a peak of approximately 90 beats/minute) and rate-pressure product (to a peak of approximately 12,000), with a small (non-significant) reduction of systolic and diastolic blood pressure. The addition of an additional 0.28 mg/kg produces a significant increment of heart-rate and blood pressure above that achieved at low dose [16].

However, despite coronary steal rather than increased workload being looked upon as the primary mechanism of action of this agent, greater hemodynamic responses appear to correlate with higher probabilities of a positive test. Thus, using a low-dose [0.56 mg/kg] protocol, Picano recorded a heart-rate increment from 73 ± 14 to 102 ± 16 in patients with true-positive findings, which significantly exceeded that in patients with false negative test results, and a similar difference was apparent for the rate-pressure product [22]. The greater hemodynamic response at positive tests may be a marker of optimal vasodilator effect, or represent a direct role for increased cardiac workload during dipyridamole stress.

The hemodynamic responses to adenosine appear to be dose-dependent, with an increment of blood-pressure and rate-pressure product in patients studied using a higher dose protocol [19,20]. Again, however, the hemodynamic changes are less than those usually associated with dobutamine or exercise stress.

5.1.4 *Side-effects of Dipyridamole and Adenosine*

As dipyridamole and adenosine are effectively the same agent, they have a similar side-effect profile. In general, as adenosine is more potent, its side-effects are more intense and frequent than those of dipyridamole, though of shorter duration.

The side-effect profile of high-dose dipyridamole echocardiography has been studied in over 10,000 patients [23]. Significant sequellae (including both major complications and dose-limiting side-effects) occurred in 113 patients (1.2%). Major adverse reactions, including myocardial infarction, pulmonary edema and malignant arrhythmias, occurred in 7 patients (0.07%), comparable to the experience reported for dipyridamole thallium imaging [5]. Five of these events were associated with the presence of myocardial ischemia, unrecognised by inexperienced operators, but the development of side-effects was otherwise unpredictable. Of the dose-limiting side-effects, the most frequent were due to ischemia, hypotension, bronchospasm and bradycardias (including complete heart block). Despite their relative rarity, deaths have been reported from these complications [5], so that dipyridamole and adenosine stress are contraindicated in patients with untreated atrioventricular block, and bronchospastic disorders. Patients with chronic obstructive airways disease who have no or minimal airways reactivity, and can tolerate the cessation of theophylline-containing compounds, may undergo the test.

About two-thirds of patients studied with the high-dose dipyridamole

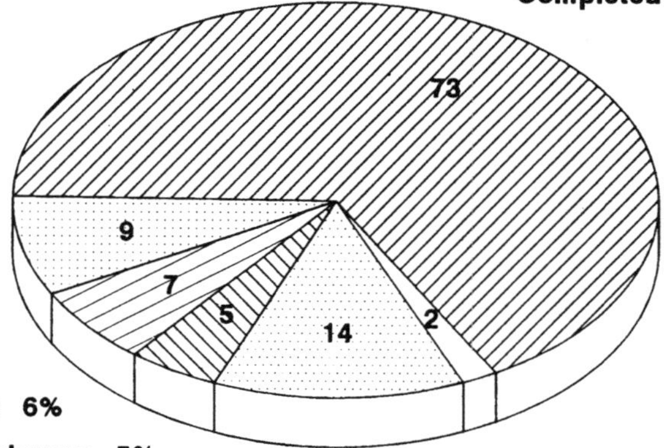

Figure 5.3. End-points of high-dose adenosine stress in 97 patients with and without coronary disease [20].

protocol experience minor side-effects, which reflect the systemic vasodilator effects of the compound, including flushing and headache [16]. However, minor side-effects rarely preclude completion of the study, partly because the infusion is completed before they become evident. These symptoms usually resolve spontaneously, but if their nature or severity warrants active treatment, the administration of aminophylline usually provides rapid relief. Nitrates are useful for relieving subendocardial ischemia, coronary spasm and angina due to increased oxygen demand. As with dobutamine echocardiography protocols, the ability to visualize the onset and severity of ischemia "on-line" enables the early recognition and treatment of ischemia.

Most patients undergoing adenosine stress develop some form of side-effect [19]; in our experience [20], side-effects prevented about a third of patients from achieving the peak dose (Figure 5.3). Qualitatively, these correspond to those experienced during dipyridamole stress, although chest discomfort (possibly due to a direct algogenic effect of adenosine) and dyspnea (which appears to be caused by a first-pass effect in the lungs) are more frequent. Cessation of the infusion is usually the only treatment required for side-effects.

5.1.5 *Accuracy of vasodilator stress testing*

Although chest pain and ST segment changes may be provoked by dipyridamole or adenosine stress, these have generally been found to be neither sensitive nor specific (see Chapter 6). As in the case of dobutamine, some form of imaging should be combined with vasodilator stress testing.

Studies addressing the accuracy of vasodilator stress echocardiography for the identification of coronary artery disease are summarized in Table 5.1 [15,16,19–22,24–32]. This table demonstrates that the sensitivity of dipyridamole stress echocardiography for the detection of coronary artery disease demonstrates significant variability between studies. As in the previous chapters on exercise and dobutamine stresses, this heterogeneity reflects differences in the definition of "significant" disease, different stress protocols, anti-anginal drug therapy, and patient selection. Most studies of dipyridamole stress echocardiography have utilized a criterion of >70% stenosis to denote significant coronary stenoses – as discussed in Chapter 2, use of this cutoff tends to enhance sensitivity, which may be lower if the test is challenged with the detection of milder stenoses (>50%). However, the variability in the results expressed in Table 5.1 occurs between studies with the same cutoff, and the test has an excellent specificity in all studies, which is inconsistent with bias introduced by a conservative criterion of disease (which inflates sensitivity at the cost of impaired specificity).

The use of the low dose (0.56 mg/kg) protocol is associated with sensitivities ranging from 56 to 82%, generally lower than those reported with the high dose regimen, which range from 58 to 94%. Similar results have even been obtained with oral dipyridamole stress [15], although the sensitivity recorded in that series may have been colored by a high prevalence of multivessel disease and the inclusion of patients with myocardial infarction. Again, however, heterogeneous results occur even in those patients tested using the same regimen.

The sensitivity of dipyridamole stress echocardiography is significantly compromised by anti-anginal drugs – beta-blockers, calcium antagonists and combination therapy [33]. The majority of subjects studied in Table 5.1 were performed off anti-anginal therapy, and the series characterized by the lowest sensitivity involved cessation of therapy for four half-lives. Thus, while anti-anginal therapy may account for low sensitivity of the test in clinical practice, it does not explain the heterogeneity of the findings in these series.

As was seen in earlier chapters, the greatest source of variability pertains to differences in study populations. The inclusion of patients with myocardial infarction, and high prevalence of multivessel coronary disease may inflate the sensitivity of any test, and multivessel disease is especially prevalent in many of the reported dipyridamole echocardiography studies – largely a reflection of the referral of patients with more extensive coronary disease to tertiary referral centers. Indeed, the sensitivity of dipyridamole echocardiography for single vessel coronary disease (Table 5.1) shows most results to be in the 50% range, even with optimal (transesophageal) imaging. The ability of standard dose dipyridamole stress to induce ischemia in patients with single vessel disease has been specifically examined by Kern [34], who confirmed that, even in the presence of a good coronary hyperemic response, only 3 of 13 patients developed regional dysfunction consistent with ischemia.

A variant of the standard vasodilator stress protocol is to combine the test with exercise [27,29] or atropine [30], which offers a greater cardiac

Table 5.1. Sensitivity and specificity of echocardiography with vasodilator stress.

Author	Ref	n	Stress technique	"Significant" stenosis dia	Multivessel (% all CAD)
Cohen	15	50	Dipy 400 mg po	>70%	28 (78%)
Picano	16	93	Dipy 0.84 mg/kg*	>70%	48 (67%)
Zoghbi	19	33	Ad 0.14 mcg/kg/min*	>75%	11 (55%)
Marwick	20	97	Ad 0.18 mcg/kg/min*	>50%	28 (47%)
Mazeika	21	55	Dipy 1.00 mg/kg*	>70%	30 (75%)
Picano	22	66	Dipy 0.56 mg/kg	>70%	20 (40%)
Masini	24	83	Dipy 0.84 mg/kg*	>70%	24 (62%)
Picano	25	445	Dipy 0.84 mg/kg*	>50%	119 (46%)
Massa	26	52	Dipy 0.84 mg/kg*	>70%	12 (23%)
Picano	27	33	Dipy 0.84 mg/kg + ex	>50%	8 (33%)
Agati	28	42	Dipy 0.60 mg/kg	>75%	22 (76%)
Labowitz	29	48	Dipy 0.56 mg/kg + ex	>70%	26 (65%)
Pingitore	30	130	Dipy 0.84 mg/kg + atr	>50%	–
Agati	31	32	Dipy 0.84 mg/kg*	>70%	18 (75%)
Previtali	32	35	Dipy 0.84 mg/kg*	>70%	12 (43%)

* Low dose positivity permits conclusion of study before stated "peak" dose.
Ad = adenosine, atr = atropine, dia = diameter of coronary artery, Dipy = dipyridamole, reference, SVD = single vessel disease, TTE = transthoracic echocardiography.

workload than is available from dipyridamole testing alone. Both combinations may be sensitive for the detection of coronary disease in patients with false negative results by conventional approaches. The use of transesophageal echocardiography [31] results in excellent image quality, but although a good option in patients with poor transthoracic images, does not solve the fundamental problem of dipyridamole having relatively "weak" ischemic potential for diagnostic testing in patients with mild disease.

The performance of imaging in a supine position permits combination of regional functional assessment with Doppler [28,29,35,36]. Early studies demonstrated a distinction between patients with coronary disease and normal controls [28,32]. However, in a recent clinical series [36], Doppler evaluation of systolic function was not found to be useful in discriminating those with and without ischemia induced by dipyridamole echocardiography, because global function was preserved by the development of compensatory hyperkinesis in non-ischemic zones. The hemodynamic effects of dipyridamole themselves alter atrioventricular flow, thus precluding Doppler evaluation of left ventricular filling as a marker of ischemia.

Two reports have described the results of adenosine stress echocardiography [19,20]. Using a peak infusion rate of 0.14 mg/kg/min, in 73 patients with suspected or known coronary disease, Zoghbi [19] reported an overall sensitivity of 85% and a specificity of 92% for the detection of >75%

M infarctn (% all CAD)	Sensitivity – overall	Sensitivity – SVD	Specificity	Comments
16 (44%)	81% (n = 36)	88% (n = 8)	93% (n = 14)	
17 (24%)	74% (n = 72)	50% (n = 12)	100% (n = 21)	
Excluded	60% (n = 20)	30% (n = 9)	92% (n = 13)	
Excluded	58% (n = 59)	52% (n = 31)	87% (n = 38)	Consecutive group
18 (45%)	40% (n = 40)	0% (n = 10)	93% (n = 15)	
9 (18%)	56% (n = 50)	37% (n = 30)	100% (n = 16)	Typical angina (79%)
15 (38%)	79% (n = 39)	–	93% (n = 44)	Females only
0 (0%)	96% (n = 256)	56% (n = 137)	96% (n = 135)	Off treatment
9 (17%)	90% (n = 52)	–	–	PTCA candidates
10 (42%)	88% (n = 24)	–	89% (n = 9)	
Excluded	82% (n = 29)	–	100% (n = 13)	
–	64% (n = 33)	–	80% (n = 15)	On treatment
–	87% (n = 94)	–	94% (n = 34)	Atr in negative DET
9 (38%)	92% (n = 24)	67% (n = 6)	100% (n = 8)	TTE not feasible
1 (4%)	57% (n = 28)	31% (n = 16)	100% (n = 7)	

DET = dipyridamole echo test, ex = exercise, M infarctn = myocardial infarction, Ref =

stenoses. However, the sensitivity was only 60% in 35 patients with a normal baseline electrocardiogram. Our experience is similar [20]; in 100 non-infarct patients studied with a high-dose protocol (0.18 mg/kg/min), the sensitivity of adenosine echocardiography was 56%.

5.1.6 *Indices of Coronary Disease Severity by Vasodilator Echocardiography*

Just as coronary disease is not an "all or none" phenomenon, the echocardiographic findings show a spectrum of changes in the dimensions of time-course, extent and severity [10]. More severe disease in the vessel supplying an ischemic region generally correlates with a more severe wall motion disturbance, and multi-vessel disease usually corresponds with more extensive areas of ischemia. The time until the onset of regional asynergy corresponds to the "ischemia-free" time at exercise testing. Hence, an early positive response at "standard dose" (0.56 mg/kg) correlates with multivessel disease [16,21], with worse prognosis [37], and with a lower ischemic threshold at exercise testing [38]. In addition to this "time co-ordinate", there is also a "space co-ordinate" [10] relating to the extent of coronary disease. Both considerations give an index of the physiologic significance of coronary disease.

5.1.7 *Selection of the Optimal Pharmacologic Stress – Dobutamine vs Dipyridamole*

In patients who cannot exercise, the above sections demonstrate that favorable clinical experience has been reported with both dobutamine and vasodilator stress echocardiography. Insofar as the contraindications of each test vary, the choice of stress may be individualized to each patient; those with hypertension or arrhythmias should undergo a vasodilator rather than an inotropic stress, and patients with bronchospasm or conduction disorders should be submitted for dobutamine testing. Most patients do not have these contraindications, however, and for this majority, few data are available to select the optimal stress. Comparison of the efficacy of the stressors in separate studies is not reasonable, given the extrinsic influences upon test accuracy, apparent in tables 4.1 and 5.1. Thus, the choice of optimal stress for provoking ischemia should preferably be based on a comparison between the agents in the same patients, under the same conditions.

Previtali [33] compared dipyridamole (0.84 mg/kg) and dobutamine (40 mcg/kg/min) stresses in a group of 35 patients with chest pain and suspected coronary artery disease. In the 12 with multivessel disease, both dobutamine and dipyridamole tests had a sensitivity of 92%. In 16 patients with single-vessel disease, dobutamine had a 50% sensitivity, compared with 31% for dipyridamole (p = NS). The specificity of both tests was 100% in 7 patients without coronary disease. This small study, in a selected group, suggested that the tests were comparable, with a possible advantage for dobutamine in detecting patients with milder disease. In 25 patients with coronary disease, studied by Martin [39], a significantly higher level of sensitivity was obtained with dobutamine (76%) than adenosine and dipyridamole (40% and 56%, respectively). This benefit was circumscribed by a significantly lower level of specificity with dobutamine (60%), compared with adenosine (93%). Dobutamine was the best tolerated agent.

We prospectively studied 97 non-infarct patients with suspected coronary disease, using adenosine (0.18 mg/kg) and dobutamine (40 mcg/kg/min) stresses [20]. Both protocols were terminated because of side-effects in about 30% of patients; but all were reversible and no serious complications occurred. There was no significant difference between the tests in terms of patient preference. Dobutamine imposed a significantly greater workload on the heart (Figure 5.4). In 62 patients with significant coronary disease (defined by the quantitation of >50% stenosis in a major epicardial vessel), the sensitivity of dobutamine echocardiography was 84%, compared with 56% for adenosine echocardiography ($p < 0.001$). This difference was more prominent in the 32 patients with single-vessel disease (81% vs 50%, $p < 0.01$) than in those with multivessel disease (87% vs 63%, $p = 0.07$). The specificity of dobutamine echocardiography was 82%, and that of adenosine echocardiography was 92% (p = NS). This larger study confirms that for the diagnosis of coronary disease, dobutamine is more sensitive than vasodilator

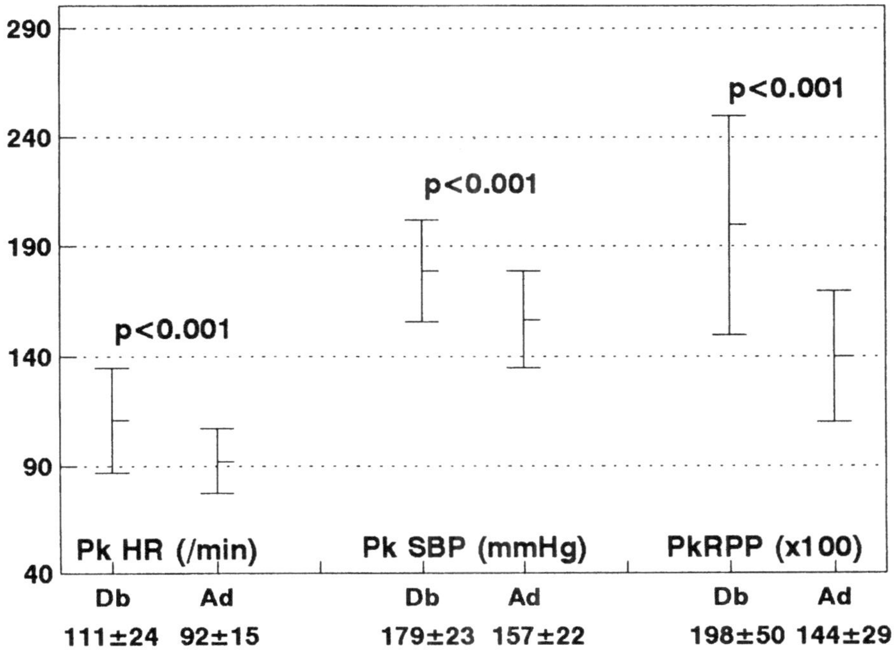

Figure 5.4. Heart-rate (HR), systolic blood pressure (SBP) and rate-pressure product (RPP) responses at peak effect (Pk) during dobutamine and adenosine stress in 97 patients with suspected coronary disease. Studies were performed under the same conditions and resting hemodynamic parameters were equivalent.

echocardiography, especially in those with milder disease. Thus, we believe that for diagnostic (not necessarily prognostic) purposes, dobutamine is the optimal non-exercise stress.

5.1.8 *Use of Dipyridamole in Preference to Exercise Stress – Is It Justified?*

As in the case of dobutamine (Chapter 4), many patients considered for dipyridamole echocardiography could potentially undergo exercise stress. In these subjects, dipyridamole has been recommended as a preferable test because of its higher feasibility, better image quality, lack of reliance on image digitization, ability to offer peak images, and stepwise protocol [40]. However, the issue must be decided on the basis of the comparitive accuracy of the tests, performed in the same patients and under the same circumstances – unfortunately, few such data exist.

Dipyridamole and exercise stress echocardiography have been compared by Picano [41]. Of 55 patients, dipyridamole studies were feasible in 100%, compared with 73% of exercise studies ($p < 0.01$). However, the latter success rate is lower than reported from most recent exercise echocardiography studies (Chapter 3), and may to an extent reflect the interpretation of the studies from video tape rather than a digitized quad-screen display. Among 40 patients in whom both studies were interpretable, the sensitivity (72% and 76%) and specificity (100% and 87%) of dipyridamole and exercise echocardiography were comparable. These results should be tempered by considerations regarding the study group; 18 of 34 patients with coronary disease had multivessel disease, stenoses of >70% diameter were considered significant, and no patients had moderate stenoses. On these grounds, the levels of sensitivity achieved are also less than might be expected from recent exercise echocardiography studies. The comparability of vasodilator stress with exercise stress has therefore not been established in an unselected group without myocardial infarction and with a wide spectrum of coronary disease severity.

5.2 Ergonovine Stress Testing

Patients with anginal symptoms, in whom stress testing and coronary angiography have been negative, are sometimes suspected of suffering from coronary spasm. Spasm may occur following prolonged hyperventilation, or may be provoked by ergonovine injection [42]. In either case, ischemia caused by coronary spasm may become evident at echocardiography as regional left ventricular dysfunction. The usual hyperventilation protocol involves 5 minutes of deep, rapid breathing, followed by 10 minutes of echocardiographic imaging. Ergonovine is administered in a step-wise protocol, involving boluses of 0.025 mg, doubled every 10 minutes until attainment of a dose of 0.4 mg, ischemia, or limiting side-effects (hypertension or nausea). This test should not be performed in patients with previous infarction or documented myocardial ischemia, and has the potential hazard of producing severe or prolonged ischemia.This stress has not met with wide acceptance in the echocardiography laboratory, and our own preference is to perform it in the angiography laboratory, with direct imaging of the spasm, and the ability to locally infuse nitrates and open the vessel mechanically, should complications arise.

References

1. Knabb RM, Gidday JM, Ely SW, Rubio R, Berne RM. Effects of dipyridamole on myocardial adenosine and active hyperemia. Am J Physiol 1984;247:H804–H810.
2. Klabunde RE. Dipyridamole inhibition of adenosine metabolism in human blood. Eur J Pharmacol 1983;9:21–6.
3. Wilson RF, White CW. Intracoronary papaverine: An ideal coronary vasodilator for studies of the coronary circulation in conscious humans. Circulation 1986;73:444–51.
4. Wilson RF, Wyche K, Christensen BV, Zimmer S, Laxson DD. Effects of adenosine on human coronary arterial circulation. Circulation 1990;82:1595–606.

5. Ranhosky A, Kempthorne-Rawson J. The safety of intravenous dipyridamole thallium myocardial perfusion imaging. Circulation 1990;81:1205–9.
6. Wendt VE, Sundermeyer JF, Denbakker PB, Bing RJ. The relationship between coronary blood flow, myocardial oxygen consumption and cardiac work as influenced by persantin. Am J Cardiol 1962;9:449–55.
7. Wilcken DEL, Paolini HJ, Eickens E. Evidence for intravenous dipyridamole producing a "coronary steal" effect in the ischaemic myocardium. Aust NZ J Med 1971;1:8–10.
8. Picano E. Dipyridamole echocardiography test: Historical background and physiological basis. Eur Heart J 1989;10:365–76.
9. Albro PC, Gould KL, Westcott RJ, Hamilton GV, Ritchie JL, Williams DL. Non-invasive assessment of coronary stenoses by myocardial imaging during pharmacologic coronary vasodilation. III Clinical trial. Am J Cardiol 1978;42:751–60.
10. Picano E, Lattanzi F. Dipyridamole echocardiography: A new diagnostic window on coronary artery disease. Circulation 1991;83(Suppl III):19–26.
11. Gross GJ, Warltier DC. Coronary steal in four models of single or multiple vessel obstruction in dogs. Am J Cardiol 1981;48:84–92.
12. Marwick T, Torelli J, Underwood D, MacIntyre WJ. Metabolic evidence of ischemia following high- and low-dose dipyridamole stress [abstract]. J Nucl Med 1992;33:866.
13. Smits P, Corstens FH, Aengevaeren WR, Wackers FJ, Thien T. False negative dipyridamole thallium-201 myocardial imaging after caffeine infusion. J Nucl Med 1991;32:1538–41.
14. Brown BG, Josephson MA, Petersen RB *et al.* Intravenous dipyridamole combined with isometric handgrip for near maximal acute increase in coronary flow in patients with coronary artery disease. Am J Cardiol 1981;48:1077–85.
15. Cohen JL, Greene TO, Alston JR, Wilchford SD, Kim CS. Usefulness of oral dipyridamole digital echocardiography for detecting coronary artery disease. Am J Cardiol 1989;64:385–6.
16. Picano E, Lattanzi F, Massini M, Distante A, L'Abbate A. High dose dipyridamole echocardiography test in effort angina pectoris. J Am Coll Cardiol 1986;8:848–54.
17. Nishimura S, Mahmarian JJ, Boyce TM, Verani MS. Quantitative thallium-201 single-photon emission computed tomography during maximal pharmacologic coronary vasodilation with adenosine for assessing coronary artery disease. J Am Coll Cardiol 1991;18:736–45.
18. Nguyen T, Heo J, Ogilby JD, Iskandrian AS. Single-photon emission computed tomography with thallium-201 during adenosine-induced coronary hyperemia: Correlation with coronary arteriography, exercise thallium imaging and two-dimensional echocardiography. J Am Coll Cardiol 1990;16:1375–83.
19. Zoghbi WA, Cheirif J, Kleiman NS, Verani MS, Trakhtenbroit A. Diagnosis of ischemic heart disease with adenosine echocardiography. J Am Coll Cardiol 1991;18:1271–9.
20. Marwick T, Willemart B, D'Hondt AM *et al.* Selection of the optimal non-exercise stress for the evaluation of ischemic regional myocardial dysfunction and malperfusion: Comparison of dobutamine and adenosine using echocardiography and Tc-99 m MIBI Single Photon Emission Computed Tomography. Circulation 1993;87:345–54.
21. Mazeika P, Nihoyannopoulos P, Joshi J, Oakley CM. Uses and limitations of high dose dipyridamole stress echocardiography for evaluation of coronary artery disease. Br Heart J 1992;67:144–9.
22. Picano E, Distante A, Masini M, Morales MA, Lattanzi F, L'Abbate A. Dipyridamole echocardiography test in effort angina pectoris. Am J Cardiol 1985;56:452–6.
23. Picano E, Marini C, Pirelli S *et al.* Safety of intravenous high-dose dipyridamole echocardiography. Am J Cardiol 1992;70:252–8.

26. Massa D, Pirelli S, Gara E *et al.* Exercise testing and dipyridamole echocardiography test before and 48h after successful coronary angioplasty: Prognostic implications. Eur Heart J 1989;10(Suppl G):13–7.
27. Picano E, Lattanzi F, Masini M, Distante A, L'Abbate A. Usefulness of the dipyridamole-exercise echocardiography test for diagnosis of coronary artery disease. Am J Cardiol 1988;62:67–70.
28. Agati L, Arata L, Neja CP *et al.* Usefulness of dipyridamole-Doppler test for diagnosis of coronary artery disease. Am J Cardiol 1990;65:829–34.
29. Labovitz AJ, Pearson AC, Chaitman BR. Doppler and two-dimensional echocardiographic assessment of left ventricular function before and after intravenous dipyridamole stress testing for detection of coronary artery disease. Am J Cardiol 1988;62:1180–5.
30. Pingitore A, Picano E, Kozakova M *et al.* Enhanced sensitivity for detection of coronary artery disease by addition of atropine to dipyridamole echocardiography [abstract]. Circulation 1992;85:I–863.
31. Agati L, Renzi M, Sciomer S *et al.* Transesophageal dipyridamole echocardiography for diagnosis of coronary artery disease. J Am Coll Cardiol 1992;19:765–70.
32. Previtali M, Lanzarini L, Ferrario M, Tortorici M, Mussini A, Montemartini C. Dobutamine versus dipyridamole echocardiography in coronary artery disease. Circulation 1991;83(Suppl III):27–31.
33. Lattanzi F, Picano E, Bolognese L *et al.* Inhibition of dipyridamole-induced ischemia by antianginal therapy in humans: Correlation with exercise echocardiography. Circulation 1991;83:1256–62.
34. Kern MJ, Pearson AC, Labovitz AJ *et al.* Effects of pharmacologic coronary hyperemia on echocardiographic left ventricular function in patients with single vessel coronary disease. J Am Coll Cardiol 1989;13:1042–51.
35. Grayburn PA, Popma JL, Pryor SL, Walker BS, Simon TR, Smitherman TC. Comparison of dipyridamole Doppler echocardiography to thallium-201 imaging and quantitative coronary arteriography in the assessment of coronary artery disease. Am J Cardiol 1989;63:1315–20.
36. Mazeika P, Nihoyannopoulos P, Joshi J, Oakley CM. Evaluation of dipyridamole-Doppler echocardiography for detection of myocardial ischemia and coronary artery disease. Am J Cardiol 1991;68:478–84
37. Picano E, Severi S, Michelassi C *et al.* Prognostic importance of dipyridamole echocardiography test in coronary artery disease. Circulation 1989;80:450–7.
38. Picano E, Lattanzi F, Masini M, Distante A, L'Abbate A. Different degrees of ischemic threshold stratified by the dipyridamole echocardiography test. Am J Cardiol 1987;59:71–3.
39. Martin TW, Seaworth JF, Johns JP, Pupa LE, Condos WR. Comparison of adenosine, dipyridamole and dobutamine in stress echocardiography. Ann Intern Med 1992;116:190–6.
40. Picano E. Stress echocardiography – From pathophysiological toy to diagnostic tool. Circulation 1992;85:1604–12.
41. Picano E, Lattanzi F, Masini M, Distante A, L'Abbate A. Comparison of the high-dose dipyridamole echocardiography test and exercise two-dimensional echocardiography for diagnosis of coronary artery disease. Am J Cardiol 1987;59:539–54.
42. Previtali M, Ardissino D, Barberis P, Panciroli C, Chimienti M, Salerno JA. Hyperventilation and ergonovine tests in Prinzmetal's variant angina pectoris in man. Am J Cardiol 1989;63:17–20.

6. Comparison of Exercise and Pharmacologic Stress Echocardiography and Electrocardiography

T. MARWICK and J-M. DETRY

The provocation of ST segment depression in response to increased cardiac work is accepted as the simplest and most widely used test for the documentation of myocardial ischemia [1]. These phenomena reflect changes in the polarity of (usually subendocardial) segments, based upon ischemia-induced disturbances in the electrical state of individual myocytes [2], and depend to some extent on the location and extent of ischemia. While the stress electocardiogram (ECG) reflects the electrical manifestation of ischemia, its ability to accurately identify this may be clouded by the development of similar ECG patterns with non-ischemic processes. These influences contrast with the sensitivity and specificity of the mechanical sequelae of ischemia, identified by echocardiography.

Comparisons between the exercise ECG and exercise echocardiography may be made on the basis of their accuracy for the diagnosis of coronary disease, their relative abilities to functionally assess disease, and their prognostic implications. This chapter will primarily address the issue of accuracy. In order to deal with the limitations posed by making this comparison in the wide spectrum of patients studied, the population will be divided into three groups: those with an interpretable ECG who are able to exercise maximally, patients with an uninterpretable ECG (due to left ventricular hypertrophy, left bundle branch block, digitalis effect etc), and those able to exercise only submaximally, or who are unable to exercise. In a recent review [3] of over 1800 patients attending the exercise laboratory of a tertiary referral center over 1 year, these groups were roughly evenly represented (Figure 6.1). The comparison between the stress ECG and stress echocardiography has different implications in each group, and will be analyzed separately.

6.1 Test Selection in Active Patients with an Interpretable ECG

6.1.1 *Current Status of the Exercise ECG*

Patients with chest pain are usually referred for exercise testing in order to confirm or exclude the diagnosis of coronary artery disease. The accuracy of 147 consecutively published studies of exercise testing was recently reviewed by Gianrossi [4]. Sensitivity and specificity were found to vary widely (from

T.H. Marwick, Stress Echocardiography, 95–111.

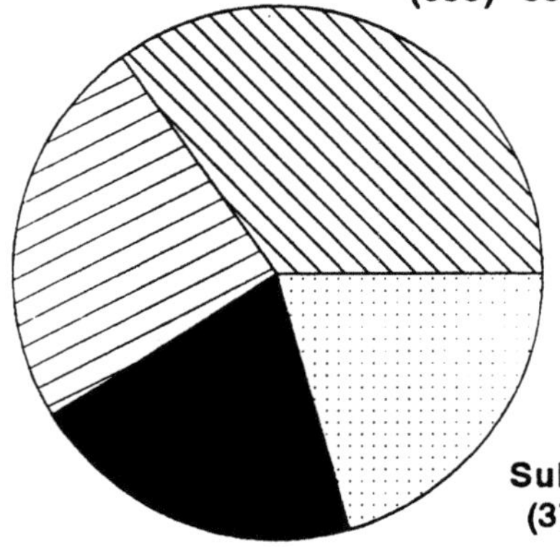

Figure 6.1. Proportion of patients with interpretable ECG and maximal exercise, uninterpretable ECG, submaximal exercise and inability to exercise, among 1814 unselected patients referred for stress testing. Reproduced with permission of Acta Clinica Belgica.

20–100%), reflecting variations in patient selection and exercise testing methodology. Even accepting these variations, the mean sensitivity and specificity were respectively 68 ± 16% and 77 ± 17%. In a series of 8 studies, selected by Detrano and Froelicher [5] on the grounds of having clinically representative populations with minimal referral bias and no review bias, the average sensitivity and specificity were 71% and 73%. This modest level of accuracy may reflect a negative influence from some subgroups with particularly poor results using the exercise ECG (discussed further in a later section of this chapter).

Attempts have been made to improve on these reported levels of accuracy, by inclusion of non-ST segment data from the exercise ECG, as well as data from the non-ECG components of the exercise test. The efficacy of incorporation of R wave amplitude [6] and heart rate data [7] into the ST analysis has been disputed [8,9]. Other authors have attained more accurate results by combining ECG data (ST depression, ST slope, R wave amplitude) with heart-rate response and exercise duration on the treadmill [10,11], or with workload on the bicycle [12]. In the latter study of 387 male patients, the use of a multivariate approach increased the sensitivity of the ECG exercise test to 82%, compared with 64% using ST segment criteria alone. The specificity was 92% with the multivariate, and 82% using ST segment interpretation. Use of this multivariate approach at another center confirmed this high level of specificity, together with enhancement of sensitivity from 70% to 84% [13].

6.1.2 *Comparisons of Exercise ECG and Exercise Echocardiography*

While the reported levels of accuracy of the exercise ECG are inferior to the 80–85% sensitivity and specificity results reported in recent exercise echocardiography studies (Chapter 3), a proper comparison between the exercise ECG and exercise echocardiography requires that both tests be performed in the same group of patients. This study design may necessitate the relocation of electrodes (usually V_2 and V_5) away from the parasternal and apical echocardiographic windows, with the possibility of an adverse effect on the accuracy of the stress ECG. Nine studies [14–23] comparing immediate post-treadmill or peak- (bicycle) exercise echocardiography with the ST segment response of the exercise ECG in the same patients are summarized in Table 6.1. The results show some heterogeneity, but generally display superiority of exercise echocardiography over the ST segment interpretation in both sensitivity and specificity. These results may to an extent be colored by the study population, especially in the larger, clinical series – patients are more likely to have been referred for echocardiography in the presence of an equivocal, or clinically inconsistent ECG result, and this finding is likely to remain negative during the exercise echocardiography test, too. Nonetheless, greater sensitivity has also been recorded in an unselected population. The inferiority of the exercise ECG with respect to specificity again reflects studies involving a comparison in all patients, including those whose ECG might otherwise have been classed as uninterpretable. Indeed, in our experience [21], once patients with non-diagnostic results were excluded, the specificity of the exercise ECG rose from 47% to 74%, becoming comparable to that of echocardiography (87%, p = NS). Interestingly, exclusion of patients with non-diagnostic ECG results did not alter the superiority of the echocardiogram with respect to sensitivity (Figure 6.2). These data support the conclusion that exercise echocardiography enhances the accuracy of the exercise ECG for the diagnosis of coronary disease, predominantly by providing greater sensitivity for its detection.

The greater sensitivity of exercise echocardiography than the exercise ECG is not surprising, as ST segment changes are a later occurrence in the "ischemic cascade" than are regional wall motion changes [24]. Indeed, the same enhancement of accuracy was demonstrated in early data examining the value of combining thallium imaging with the exercise test [25]. Nonetheless, the adequacy of the exercise ECG in these studies has been questioned, partly because the reported sensitivities are less than those in the above reviews of ECG exercise testing, and also because the comparison of echocardiography with the ST segment evaluation neglects other aspects of the ECG and exercise data which may be important. One study has approached this issue in a preliminary form [26], by comparing exercise echocardiography with the multivariate score of Detry [12]. In 59 patients with coronary disease, the sensitivity of this score (78%) was not significantly less than that of exercise echocardiography (90%), but the latter was more sensitive than was

Table 6.1. Comparison of sensitivity and specificity of exercise stress echocardiography and

Author	Ref	n	Method - stress	Method - ECG	Sensitivity - echo	Sensitivity - ECG
Morganroth	14	30	Supine bike	12-lead	63% (n = 19)	63% (n = 19)
Maurer	15	36	Treadmill	II, V5	83% (n = 23)	52% (n = 23)
Limacher	16	73	Treadmill	12-lead	91% (n = 56)	86% (n = 56)
Armstrong	17	59	Treadmill	3-lead	80% (n = 44)	59% (n = 32)
Ryan	18	64	Treadmill	3-lead	78% (n = 40)	60% (n = 35)
Galanti	19	53	Upright bike	12-lead	93% (n = 27)	78% (n = 27)
Crouse	20	228	Treadmill	NS	97% (n = 175)	51% (n = 175)
Marwick	21	82	Treadmill	12-lead	87% (n = 54)	63% (n = 40)
Ryan	22	309	Upright bike	3-lead	91% (n = 211)	40% (n = 131)
Hecht	23	180	Supine bike	12-lead	93% (n = 137)	52% (n = 137)

Echo = exercise echocardiogram, ECG = exercise ECG, MI = myocardial infarction, ref =

of ST segment analysis alone (63%, $p = 0.01$). The tests did not differ significantly in specificity (Figure 6.3). More data are needed before it can be concluded that these newer approaches to exercise ECG testing produce comparable data to exercise echocardiography. In particular, to become

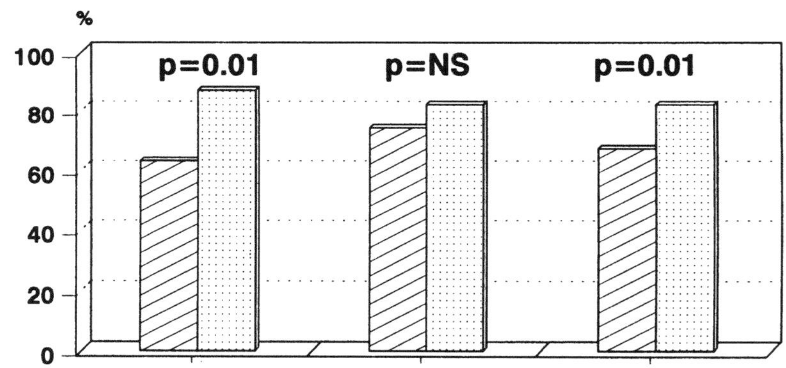

	Sensitivity	Specificity	Accuracy
Exercise ECG	63	74	67
Exercise echo	87	82	82

Exercise ECG   Exercise echo

Excluding; postMI pts, nondiagnostic ECG negative tests at submax exercise.

Figure 6.2. Sensitivity, specificity and accuracy of exercise echocardiography (echo) and exercise ECG [21] after exclusion of patients with non-diagnostic echo (negative test at a submaximal exercise) or ECG (uninterpretable ECG or negative submaximal exercise).

the exercise ECG for the detection of coronary artery disease.

Specificity - echo	Specificity - ECG	Exclusions
91% (n = 11)	91% (n = 11)	MI patients
92% (n = 13)	77% (n = 13)	MI patients
88% (n = 17)	94% (n = 17)	None (n = 29 pts with MI)
87% (n = 15)	89% (n = 9)	MI patients
100% (n = 24)	50% (n = 22)	Abnormal resting WM
96% (n = 26)	65% (n = 26)	Abnormal resting WM
64% (n = 53)	62% (n = 53)	MI's not specified
82% (n = 28)	74% (n = 23)	MI patients, non-diagnostic ECG
78% (n = 98)	89% (n = 74)	None
86% (n = 43)	86% (n = 43)	None

reference number, WM = wall motion.

widely applicable, a multivariate exercise score must be developed with treadmill exercise testing.

6.1.3 *Comparison of the Exercise ECG with Non-exercise Echocardiography*

The relative technical ease of pharmacologic stress echocardiography has led to interest in the performance of non-exercise stress in patients who are otherwise able to exercise. In this context, stress echocardiography has retained its superiority over the stress ECG alone (Table 6.2). With respect to dobutamine [27–32], the only exceptions to the greater sensitivity of echocardiography over the exercise ECG related to those individuals undergoing a submaximal dobutamine study [32]. For dipyridamole [33–36], there is some variation in the recorded sensitivity of stress echocardiography (see Chapter 5), with one report suggesting that the exercise ECG is more sensitive [36]. With both stressors, in relatively small numbers of patients, the specificity of pharmacologic stress echocardiography exceeded that of the exercise ECG.

6.2 Use of Stress Echocardiography in Subgroups Where the Stress ECG is Unreliable

6.2.1 *Patients in Whom the Resting ECG Shows Repolarization Abnormalities*

Patients with left ventricular hypertrophy, left bundle branch block, digitalis therapy or sometimes prior myocardial infarction exhibit repolarization abnormalities on the resting ECG. The existence of these resting ST segment

Table 6.2. Comparison of sensitivity and specificity of pharmacologic stress echocardiography

Author	Ref	n	Comparison - stress	Method - ECG	Sensitivity - echo	Sensitivity - ECG
Palac	27	39	Db vs TML	NS	84% (n = 25)	60% (n = 25)
Hoffman	28	48	Db vs U-Bk	NS	88% (n = NS)	64% (n = 34)
Berthe	29	30	Db vs U-Bk	12-lead	85% (n = 13)	42% (n = 12)
Mazeika	30	50	Db vs TML	12-lead	78% (n = 36)	72% (n = 36)
Salustri	31	35	Db vs U-Bk	12-lead	62% (n = 26)	46% (n = 26)
Marwick	32	86	Db vs U-Bk	3-lead	54% (n = 56)	77% (n = 56)
Picano	33	66	Dipy vs U-Bk	12-lead	56% (n = 50)	62% (n = 50)
Picano	34	93	Dipy vs U-Bk	12-lead	74% (n = 72)	69% (n = 72)
Massini	35	68	Dipy vs U-Bk	12-lead	77% (n = 26)	69% (n = 26)
Mazeika	36	55	Dipy vs TML	12-lead	40% (n = 40)	80% (n = 40)

Db = dobutamine, Dipy = dipyridamole, Echo = exercise echocardiogram, ECG = exercise TML = treadmill, U-Bk = upright bicycle exercise, WM = wall motion.

changes limits the ability to discern ischemia-induced changes, and such patients are usually classified as having exercise tests which are uninterpretable for the presence of ischemia. On these grounds, it is inappropriate to compare the results of exercise echocardiography with an attempted ECG interpretation. Instead, the question must be whether exercise echocardio-

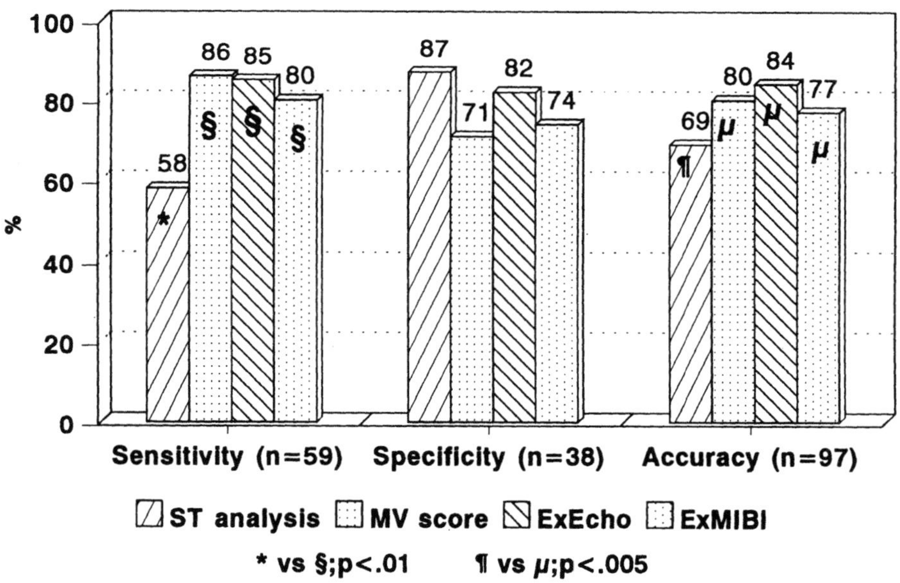

Figure 6.3. Sensitivity, specificity and accuracy of ST segment interpretation, multivariate (MV) exercise score, perfusion scintigraphy (ExMIBI) and exercise echocardiography (ExEcho) after exclusion of patients with uninterpretable ECG.

and the exercise ECG for the detection of coronary artery disease.

Specificity - echo	Specificity - ECG	Comments
86% (n = 25)	79% (n = 14)	
84% (n = NS)	85% (n = 14)	Excluded poor image quality
88% (n = 17)	73% (n = 15)	Post-MI, submaximal exercise tests
93% (n = 14)	71% (n = 14)	Excluded uninterpretable ECG
67% (n = 9)	89% (n = 9)	
83% (n = 30)	43% (n = 30)	Included submaximal Db stresses
100% (n = 16)	69% (n = 16)	
100% (n = 21)	71% (n = 21)	
93% (n = 42)	52% (n = 42)	Females, MI excluded
93% (n = 15)	67% (n = 15)	Db positivity = new/worse WMA

ECG, MI = myocardial infarction, NS = not stated, ref = reference number,

graphy is an effective test for the diagnosis of coronary disease in patients whose stress ECG is uninterpretable. The accuracy of exercise echocardiography in these situations has been confirmed in two studies. Armstrong [17] found that of 18 patients with an ambiguous ST segment response, the sensitivity of exercise echocardiography in the 12 patients with coronary artery disease was 75%, while its specificity was 100% in the 6 patients without disease. Marwick [21] reported on 34 patients with submaximal exercise capacity or uninterpretable ECG findings; the sensitivity of exercise echocardiography was 71% among 21 patients with coronary disease, and its specificity was 85%. Stress echocardiography has similarly been shown to be accurate in patients with left bundle branch block [37].

6.2.2 *Patients with Left Ventricular Hypertrophy*

The identification of coronary artery disease in patients with left ventricular hypertrophy is a frequent clinical challenge. In this condition, the accuracy of ECG stress testing is compromised [38], as also is the accuracy of myocardial perfusion imaging, which is discussed in Chapter 7.

While the role of both exercise and non-exercise stress echocardiography in the setting of left ventricular hypertrophy is still being established, standard resting echocardiography has gained acceptance as the test of choice for the definition of left ventricular hypertrophy. Ventricular dimensions are usually measured from M-mode images; septal thickness (S), ventricular end-diastolic dimension (EDD), and posterior wall (PW) thickness are measured just below mitral valve leaflet level, and left ventricular mass is calculated using the formula [39]:

$$\text{Echocardiographic LV mass (g)} = 1.04\{(S + EDD + PW)^3 - EDD^3\}.$$

To obtain left ventricular mass values consistent with necropsy data, the echocardiographic mass is corrected to give the true mass [40];

True LV mass = 0.8 (echocardiographic LV mass) + 0.6 g.

Hypertrophy may then be defined in accordance with the Framingham data, as ⩾131 g/m^2 in males, and ⩾100 g/m^2 in females [41].

The influence of left ventricular hypertrophy (defined by LV mass criteria) on the accuracy of exercise echocardiography has been examined [42] in a group of 127 patients with known coronary anatomy, who had echocardiograms of adequate quality for ventricular mass calculation (Figure 6.4). This group was separated into subgroups with (n = 69) and without left ventricular hypertrophy (n = 58). These groups had comparable clinical, exercise and angiographic features, but more excellent ("A" quality) studies were obtained in those with left ventricular hypertrophy. Wall motion abnormalities were present in 24 of the 29 patients with coronary artery disease and hypertrophy (sensitivity 83%), in contrast to 15 of the 22 patients with coronary artery disease but without hypertrophy (sensitivity 68%, p = NS). Normal ventricular function was observed in 39 of the 40 patients without coronary disease but with hypertrophy (specificity 98%), compared with 30 of 36 patients without either (specificity 83%, p = 0.05). The overall accuracies with and without left ventricular hypertrophy were 91% and 78% (p = 0.02), respectively. Moreover, exercise echocardiography was significantly more sensitive than the exercise ECG.

In summary, these results suggest that the accuracy of exercise echocardiography is not compromised in patients with left ventricular hypertrophy – indeed, the specificity was superior among those with this problem, possibly due to better image quality. In any event, stress echocardiography appears to be unique amoung the conventional non-invasive tests for coronary artery disease, as the others are significantly influenced by co-existent hypertrophy.

6.2.3 *Diagnosis of Coronary Artery Disease in Females*

The routine exercise ECG has proven to be unreliable for the diagnosis of coronary artery disease in women [43–47]; values for sensitivity range from 61 to 73%, and for specificity, from 59 to 79%. The problem of the exercise ECG in females thus pertains to lack of both sensitivity and specificity in the ST segment response. As in the case of male patients with suspected coronary artery disease, a multivariate approach (including non-ECG exercise variables), has been shown to improve both the sensitivity (59% to 70%) and specificity (77% to 93%) of detection of coronary artery disease in females [48]. Myocardial perfusion imaging has also been shown to circumvent this problem [46,47]. While use of this modality as a first-line test in all female patients is clearly not applicable from the standpoints of cost and availability, it may be useful in a sequential approach [47].

To date, two studies have compared the accuracy of stress echocardio-

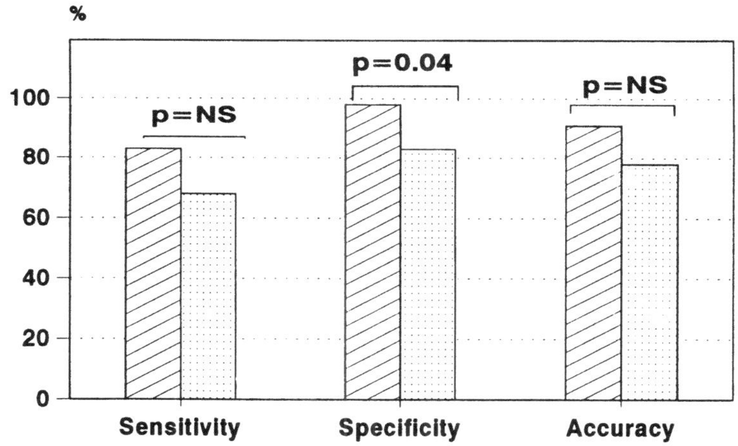

	Sensitivity	Specificity	Accuracy
LV hypertrophy	83	98	91
Normal LV mass	68	83	78

LV hypertrophy Normal LV mass

Figure 6.4. Sensitivity, specificity and accuracy of exercise echocardiography in patients with and without left ventricular hypertrophy.

graphy and stress ECG in females. In a study of 83 consecutive women presenting for evaluation of chest pain [49], the 39 with coronary disease were detected with equivalent sensitivity by high-dose dipyridamole echocardiography and the exercise ECG (79% versus 72%, p = NS). However, the 44 without significant disease were more readily recognised as being normal using dipyridamole echocardiography than with the exercise ECG (specificity 93% versus 52%, $p < 0.001$). Similar findings were reported by Sawada [50], in a group of 57 women, among whom the sensitivity and specificity of exercise echocardiography were both 86%, as compared with 29% and 83% with the exercise ECG alone. These studies indicate that stress echocardiography is a more accurate test than the stress ECG for the diagnosis of coronary artery disease in females.

6.3 Pharmacologic Stress Echocardiography versus Electrocardiography in Patients Who Are Unable to Exercise

Many patients referred for stress testing because of symptoms suggestive of coronary disease are either unable to exercise, or exercise submaximally. Patients in this group should be investigated using a non-exercise test (discussed in Chapter 4). As this group constitutes a major proportion of patients seen in routine practice (Figure 6.1), the decision as to whether pharmacologic testing may be performed with the ECG alone, or whether imaging is

Table 6.3. Comparison of sensitivity and specificity of pharmacologic stress echocardiography and ST changes at the same stress, for the detection of coronary artery disease.

Author	Ref	n	Significant stenosis	Multivessel (% al CAD)	Stress methodology	ECG leads	Sensitivity echo
Sawada	53	55	>50% dia	14 (40%)	Db to 30 mcg	3 or 12	89% (n = 35)
Cohen	54	70	>70% dia	35 (69%)	Db to 40 mcg	12	86% (n = 51)
Salustri	31	52	>50% dia	17 (46%)	Db to 40 mcg	12	54% (n = 37)
Marcowitz	55	141	>50% dia	47 (43%)	Db to 30 mcg	12	96% (n = 109)
Mazieka	30	50	>70% dia	24 (67%)	Db to 20 mcg	12	64% (n = 36)
Marwick	37	217	>50% dia	74 (52%)	Db to 40 mcg	X, Y, Z	72% (n = 142)
Picano	33	66	>70% dia	20 (40%)	Dipy 0.56 mg iv	12	56% (n = 50)
Picano	34	93	>70% dia	48 (67%)	Dipy 0.84 mg iv	12	74% (n = 72)
Massini	35	83	>70% dia	24 (61%)	Dipy 0.84 mg iv	12	79% (n = 39)
Picano	57	33	>50% dia	8 (33%)	Dipy 0.84 mg + ex	12	88% (n = 24)
Cohen	58	50	>70% dia	28 (78%)	Dipy 400 mg po	12	81% (n = 36)
Agati	59	42	>75% dia	22 (76%)	Dipy 0.60 mg iv	12	82% (n = 29)
Mazeika	36	55	>70% dia	30 (75%)	Dipy 1.00 mg iv	12	40% (n = 40)
Marwick	60	97	>50% dia	28 (47%)	Ad .18 mcg/kg/mn	X, Y, Z	58% (n = 59)
Zoghbi	61	33	>75% dia	11 (55%)	Ad .14 mcg/kg/mn	12	60% (n = 20)

Ad = adenosine, Db = dobutamine, dia = diameter of coronary artery, Dipy = dipyridamole, ex = Ref = reference.

necessarily required, has major implications with regard to workload and clinical cost.

6.3.1 *Echocardiography or ECG for Dobutamine Stress Testing*?

Dobutamine increases cardiac work in a fashion comparable to that of exercise. It might therefore be hoped that results similar to those of the exercise ECG could be available from the dobutamine ECG. Initial studies, using 5 minute increments of dobutamine, to a peak dose of 20 mcg/kg/minute, were optimistic in this respect. In a group of 75 post-infarction patients studied by Coma-Canella [51], dobutamine-induced ST depression (>1 mm) had a sensitivity of 84%, and a specificity of 64% for the detection of multivessel disease – the suboptimal specificity being ascribed to peri-infarct ischemia causing a positive test in patients with coronary disease restricted to the infarct-related artery. In a group of 90 patients (70 of whom had prolonged or unstable angina), the presence of angina and/or >1 mm ST segment depression had a sensitivity of 95% in 63 patients who had significant coronary disease [52].

Unfortunately, these results for the dobutamine stress ECG have not been replicated in studies using the usual dobutamine stress echocardiography protocols, in patients with a lower pre-test probability of coronary disease [30,31,37,53–55]. In these studies (Table 6.3), ECG sensitivities in the 25%

segment changes at the same stressechocardiography compared with ST segment

Sensitivity ST changes	Specificity echo	Specificity ST changes	Comments
23% (n = 35)	85% (n = 20)	95% (n = 20)	MI excluded
12% (n = 51)	95% (n = 19)	95% (n = 19)	MI included
24% (n = 52)	80% (n = 15)	100% (n = 15)	MI included
17% (n = 109)	66% (n = 32)	–	MI included
47% (n = 36)	93% (n = 14)	71% (n = 14)	MI included
28% (n = 131)	83% (n = 75)	94% (n = 65)	Excl non-dx ECG, MI
36% (n = 50)	100% (n = 16)	88% (n = 16)	MI included
61% (n = 72)	100% (n = 21)	86% (n = 21)	MI included
62% (n = 39)	93% (n = 44)	50% (n = 44)	Females only
75% (n = 24)	89% (n = 9)	89% (n = 9)	MI included
17% (n = 36)	93% (n = 14)	100% (n = 14)	MI included
38% (n = 29)	100% (n = 13)	100% (n = 13)	MI excluded
38% (n = 40)	93% (n = 15)	80% (n = 15)	MI included
23% (n = 57)	87% (n = 38)	90% (n = 33)	Excl non-dx ECG, MI
45% (n = 20)	92% (n = 13)	100% (n = 13)	Normal resting ECG

exercise, excl = excluded, MI = myocardial infarction, non-dx = non-diagnostic,

range have been more representative, with the exception of Mazeika's study [30], which used a longer duration of dobutamine administration, as well as being designed to identify more severe (>70%) stenoses. These studies have also shown the specificity to be in the range of 95%. Even after the exclusion of uninterpretable ECG results, in our experience in 196 patients without myocardial infarction, presenting for diagnostic angiography, the sensitivity of ≥0.1 mV ST segment depression or elevation was 28% in the 131 who had coronary disease, and its specificity was 94% [37]. Defining a positive test on the presence of either pain or significant ST segment changes increased the sensitivity to 52%, at the cost of a reduction in specificity to 67%. These findings are analogous to those of Sawada [53], in whose study the sensitivity of ST segment changes alone were enhanced from 23% to 46% by the inclusion of angina in the definition of a positive test, with a smaller fall in specificity from 95% to 90%.

The results discussed above were obtained by the application of ST segment criteria developed for use with exercise, to dobutamine testing. The pattern of low sensitivity and high specificity suggests that these criteria are not optimal for dobutamine testing. Clearly, the propensity for ECG artifact is less with pharmacologic than with exercise stress, and the possibility was considered that the criterion of ≥1 mV ST depression was not required to obtain adequate specificity with this test. We therefore performed an empiric receiver operating curve analysis (Figure 6.5) to determine whether the use

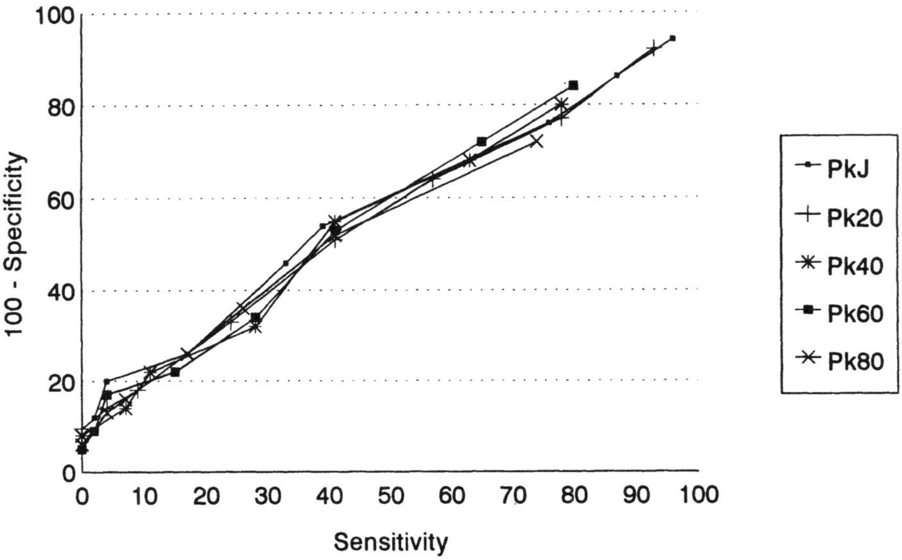

Figure 6.5. Empiric receiver operating curves for optimal degree of ST segment depression, ranging from 0 to 80 msec after the J-point.

of other ST segment criteria could enhance the accuracy of the ST segment interpretation alone [56]. One hundred and thirty-three pts with known coronary anatomy, an interpretable ECG and without previous infarction were studied. A standard dobutamine protocol (5 to 40 mcg/kg/min) was used, and ECG leads X, Y and Z were filtered and recorded digitally at the end of each stage. Using >50% diameter stenoses to define CAD, various criteria of ST segment depression (both absolute and relative to the resting state) were used to create receiver operating curves at 0–80 msec after the J-point. Conventional criteria (≥1 mm horizontal or downsloping ST depression at 60 msec after the J point) gave a sensitivity (n = 87) of 17% for the dobutamine ECG, with a specificity of 96%, and an accuracy 43%. The optimal receiver operating curve was obtained using absolute measurements of ≥0.5 mm ST depression at 80 msec after the J-point. However, although the results were better – this cutoff gave a sensitivity of 36% ($p < 0.03$ vs conventional criteria), specificity of 85%, and accuracy of 52% – they were still unsatisfactory.

Several possible explanations may underlie the heterogeneity in the observed results of dobutamine stress ECG. Discrepancies may relate in part to the use of different protocols, and in some instances, poor results for ECG sensitivity may reflect the use of extensive wall motion abnormalities (which may precede ST segment change) as a stress endpoint. However, it is most likely that the earlier, favorable results reflect use of the dobutamine ECG in populations at high risk of coronary disease [51,52]. Irrespective of the cause, the results of ST change alone are so poor that we have concluded that the combination of dobutamine with an imaging technique is essential for routine diagnostic use.

6.3.2 *Echocardiography or ECG for Vasodilator Stress Testing?*

The accuracy of the ST segment response for the diagnosis of coronary disease at dipyridamole- and adenosine-stress testing is also compared with the results of echocardiography in Table 6.3 [33–36,57–61]. After the initial proposal of dipyridamole as a stress agent, several studies showed moderately favorable levels of accuracy using dipyridamole-ECG testing [62]. As in the case of dobutamine, these results probably reflected the study population more than the efficacy of the stress for inducing ischemia.

We studied 90 patients with an ECG interpretable for ischemic changes; the sensitivity of adenosine-induced ST segment depression or elevation ($\geq$0.1 mV) was 23% in 57 patients with coronary disease, with a specificity of 90% [60]. These results were concordant with the 35% sensitivity and 100% specificity reported by Zoghbi [61].

In general, neither dipyridamole nor adenosine are particularly effective for inducing ischemic ST segment changes. We believe that some form of cardiac imaging is mandatory if these agents are selected as stressors for the detection of coronary disease in patients who are unable to exercise.

6.4 Implications – Should an Exercise Echocardiogram be Performed in All Patients with Suspected Coronary Disease?

Despite the more favorable results of stress echocardiography over stress ECG testing in many of the above subgroups, we have not made a global alteration of our practice in respect of replacing the exercise ECG. Patients undergo exercise testing for various reasons other than for the diagnosis of coronary disease, including for prognostic purposes, for evaluation of arrhythmias, and to assist in decision-making regarding coronary interventions. In these latter circumstances, the ST segment data are of secondary importance to information pertaining to exercise capacity and hemodynamic responses to exercise. Use of exercise echocardiography as a diagnostic tool in these situations may be inappropriate if these other exercise data are the most important to obtain.

The diagnostic use of the exercise stress test requires optimal accuracy in those patients with a moderate risk of coronary disease. Patients being tested at the extremes of high- or low-pretest disease probability have their post-test probability little influenced by the test result, and if studied with an exercise test, should have the procedure performed for purposes of documenting exercise capacity. The question of replacing the stress ECG with stress echocardiography therefore pertains mainly to diagnostic stress testing in patients with a moderate risk of coronary disease. This question will be addressed with respect to the groups discussed above.

In our practice, patients who cannot exercise, or who are likely to exercise submaximally, are referred for a pharmacologic stress test. The choice of echocardiography versus scintigraphy for this purpose will be discussed in Chapter 7. Nonetheless, the poor sensitivity of dobutamine, dipyridamole and adenosine stress ECG all indicate that echocardiography (or another imaging modality) is mandatory in combination with these stressors.

Patients with an uninterpretable ECG due to repolarization abnormalities should have echocardiography (or another imaging test) combined with any stress testing protocol. An argument can be made for primary use of exercise echocardiography in those in whom the exercise ECG is known to be misleading, including females and patients with mitral valve prolapse. However, we believe that more consideration needs to be given to the newer multivariate stress approaches (which benefit from objective computerized analysis), before exercise echocardiography is accepted as the primary investigation for coronary artery disease in these groups.

In patients who are able to exercise maximally, with an interpretable resting ECG, exercise echocardiography should not replace the routine exercise ECG as a first investigation. In this setting, we use echocardiography as a secondary option, if the initial exercise ECG has provided equivocal results. This strategy, involving performance of exercise echocardiography as a second test, after an initial routine exercise ECG, is analogous to the conventional application of thallium perfusion scintigraphy. The latter is recommended in situations when the initial exercise test has proven misleading or non-diagnostic (exercise-induced pain without ST segment changes), or when the exercise ECG results are at variance with the pre-test disease likelihood (for example, elderly males with typical ischemic chest pain but without typical ECG changes).

Non-invasive testing for coronary disease is not, of course, restricted to diagnostic indications. Use of the stress echocardiogram as a primary investigation is also reasonable in situations where management questions are poorly answered by the exercise ECG alone – for example, when a "culprit" vessel or the presence of multivessel disease requires definition.

References

1. Chaitman BR. The changing role of the exercise electrocardiogram as a diagnostic and prognostic test for chronic ischemic heart disease. J Am Coll Cardiol 1986;8:1195–210.
2. Becker RC, Alpert JS. Electrocardiographic ST segment depression in coronary heart disease. Am Heart J 1988;115:862–8.
3. Marwick T. Current status of non-invasive techniques for the diagnosis of myocardial ischemia. Acta Clin Belg 1992;47:1–5.
4. Gianrossi R, Detrano R, Mulvihill D *et al.* Exercise-induced ST depression in the diagnosis of coronary artery disease: A meta-analysis. Circulation 1989;80:87–98.

5. Detrano R, Froelicher VF. Exercise testing: Uses and limitations considering recent studies. Prog Cardiovasc Dis 1988;31:173–204.
6. Bonoris PE, Greenberg PS, Castellanet MJ, Ellestad MH. Significance of changes in R wave amplitudeduring treadmill stress testing: Angiographic correlation. Am J Cardiol 1978;41:846–51.
7. Kligfield P, Okin PM, Amiesen O, Wallis J, Borer RS. Correlation of the exercise ST/HR slope with anatomic and radionuclide cineangiographic findings in stable angina pectoris. Am J Cardiol 1985;56:418–21.
8. Myers J, Ahnve S, Froelicher V, Sullivan M. Spatial R wave amplitude changes during exercise: relation with left ventricular ischemia and function. J Am Coll Cardiol 1985;6:603–8.
9. Quyyumi AA, Raphael MJ, Wright C, Bealing L, Fox KM. Inability of the ST segment/heart rate slope to predict accurately the severity of coronary artery disease. Br Heart J 1984;51:395–8.
10. Hollenberg M, Budge WR, Wisneski JA, Gertz EW. Treadmill score quantifies electrocardiographic response to exercise and improves test accuracy and reproducibility. Circulation 1980;61:276–85.
11. Cohn K, Kamm B, Feteih N, Brand R, Goldschlager N. Use of treadmill score to quantify ischemic response and predict extent of coronary disease. Circulation 1979;59:286–96.
12. Detry J-M, Robert A, Luwaert RJ *et al.* Diagnostic value of computerized exercise testing in men without previous myocardial infarction. A multivariate compartmental and probabilistic approach. Eur Heart J 1985;6:227–38.
13. Deckers JW, Rensing BJ, Tyssen JG, Vincke RH, Azar AJ, Simoons ML. A Comparison of methods of analyzing exercise tests for diagnosis of coronary artery disease. Br Heart J 1989;62:438–44.
14. Morganroth J, Chen CC, David D *et al.* Exercise cross-sectional echocardiographic diagnosis of coronary artery disease. Am J Cardiol 1981;47:20–6.
15. Maurer G, Nanda NC. Two dimensional echocardiographic evaluation of exercise-induced left and right ventricular asynergy: Correlation with thallium scanning. Am J Cardiol 1981;48:720–7.
16. Limacher MC, Quinones MA, Poliner LR, Nelson JG, Winters WL, Waggoner AD. Detection of coronary artery disease with exercise two-dimensional echocardiography. Circulation 1983;67:1211–8.
17. Armstrong WF, O'Donnell J, Dillon JC, McHenry PL, Morris SN, Feigenbaum H. Complementary value of two-dimensional exercise echocardiography to routine treadmill testing. Ann Intern Med 1986;105:829–35.
18. Ryan T, Vasey CG, Presti CF, O'Donnell J, Feigenbaum H, Armstrong WF. Exercise echocardiography: Detection of coronary artery disease in patients with normal left ventricular wall motion at rest. J Am Coll Cardiol 1988;11:993–9.
19. Galanti G, Sciagra R, Comeglio M *et al.* Diagnostic accuracy of peak exercise echocardiography in coronary artery disease; Comparison with thallium-201 myocardial scintigraphy. Am Heart J 1991;122:1609–16.
20. Crouse LJ, Harbrecht JJ, Vacek JL, Rosamond TL, Kramer PH. Exercise echocardiography as a screening test for coronary artery disease and correlation with coronary arteriography. Am J Cardiol 1991;67:1213–8.
21. Marwick T, Nemec J, Pashkow FJ, Stewart WJ, Salcedo EE. Accuracy and limitations of exercise echocardiography in a routine clinical setting. J Am Coll Cardiol 1992;19:74–81.
22. Ryan T, Segar DS, Sawada SG *et al.* Detection of coronary artery disease with upright bicycle exercise echocardiography. J Am Soc Echocardiogr 1993;6:186–97.
23. Hecht HS, DeBord L, Shaw R *et al.* Digital supine bicycle stress echocardiography: A new technique for evaluating coronary disease. J Am Coll Cardiol 1993;21:950–6.
24. Upton MT, Rerych SK, Newman GE, Port S, Cobb FR, Jones RH. Detecting abnormalities in left ventricular function during exercise before angina and ST segment depression. Circulation 1980;62:341–9.

25. Ritchie JL, Trobaugh GB, Hamilton GW *et al.* Myocardial imaging with thallium-201 at rest and during exercise: Comparison with coronary arteriography and resting and stress electrocardiography. Circulation 1977;56:66–71.
26. Marwick T, D'Hondt AM, Robert AR *et al.* Accuracy of multivariate exercise score for coronary disease diagnosis: Comparison with exercise echocardiography and MIBI-SPECT [abstract]. J Am Coll Cardiol 1993;21:160A.
27. Palac RT, Coombs BJ, Kudenchuk PJ, Crane SK, Murphy ES. Two-dimensional echocardiography during dobutamine infusion - Comparison with exercise testing in evaluation of coronary disease [abstract]. Circulation 1984;70:II–184.
28. Hoffmann R, Lethen H, Kleinhans E, Flachskampf FA, Hanrath P. Comparison of bicycle and dobutamine stress echocardiography for identification of coronary artery disease [abstract]. Circulation 1991;84:II–476.
29. Berthe C, Pierard LA, Hiernaux M *et al.* Predicting the extent and location of coronary artery disease in acute myocardial infarction by echocardiography during dobutamine infusion. Am J Cardiol 1986;58:1167–72.
30. Mazieka PK, Nadazdin A, Oakley CM. Dobutamine stress echocardiography fpr detection and assessment of coronary artery disease. J Am Coll Cardiol 1992;19:1203–11.
31. Salustri A, Fioretti PR, Pozzoli MMA, McNeill AJ, Roelandt JR. Dobutamine stress echocardiography: its role in the diagnosis of coronary artery disease. Eur Heart J 1992;13:70–7.
32. Marwick T, D'Hondt A-M, Mairesse G *et al.* Should patients able to exercise undergo exercise or dobutamine echocardiography? [abstract] Eur Heart J 1993;14:454.
33. Picano E, Distante A, Masini M, Morales MA, Lattanzi F, L'Abbate A. Dipyridamole echocardiography test in effort angina pectoris. Am J Cardiol 1985;56:452–6.
34. Picano E, Lattanzi F, Massini M, Distante A, L'Abbate A. High dose dipyridamole echocardiography test in effort angina pectoris. J Am Coll Cardiol 1986;8:848–54.
35. Masini M, Picano E, Lattanzi F, Distante A, L'Abbate A. High-dose dipyridamole echocardiography test in women: Correlation with exercise-electrocardiography test and coronary arteriography. J Am Coll Cardiol 1988;12:682–5.
36. Mazeika P, Nihoyannopoulos P, Joshi J, Oakley CM. Uses and limitations of high dose dipyridamole stress echocardiography for evaluation of coronary artery disease. Br Heart J 1992;67:144–9.
37. Marwick T, D'Hondt AM, Baudhuin T *et al.* Optimal use of dobutamine stress for the detection and evaluation of coronary artery disease: Combination with echocardiography, scintigraphy or both? J Am Coll Cardiol 1993;22:159–67.
38. Harris CN, Aronow WS, Parker DP, Kaplan MA. Treadmill stress test in left ventricular hypertrophy. Chest 1973;63:353–8.
39. Devereux RB, Reichek N. Echocardiographic determination of left ventricular mass in man: Anatomic validation of the method. Circulation 1976;55:613–8.
40. Devereux RB, Alonso DR, Lutas EM *et al.* Echocardiographic assessment of left ventricular hypertrophy: comparison to necropsy findings. Am J Cardiol 1986; 57:450–8.
41. Levy D, Savage DD, Garrison RJ, Anderson KM, Kannel WB, Castelli, WP. Echocardiographic criteria for left ventricular hypertrophy: The Framingham heart study. Am J Cardiol 1987;59:956–60.
42. Torelli J, Marwick T, Nemec J *et al.* Influence of left ventricular hypertrophy on the accuracy of exercise echocardiography [abstract]. J Am Coll Cardiol 1992;19:337A.
43. Sketch MH, Mohiuddin SM, Lynch JD, Zencka AE, Runco V. Significant sex differences in the correlation of electrocardiographic exercise testing and coronary arteriograms. Am J Cardiol 1975;36:169–73.
44. Linhart JW, Laws JG, Satinsky JD. Maximum treadmill exercise electrocardiography in female patients. Circulation 1974;50:1173–8.
45. Detry J-M, Kapita BM, Cosyns J, Sottiaux B, Brasseur LA, Rousseau MF. Diagnostic value of history and maximal exercise electrocardiography in men and women suspected of heart disease. Circulation 1977;56:756–61.

46. Hung J, Chaitman BR, Lam J *et al.* Noninvasive diagnostic test choices for the evaluation of coronary artery disease in women: A multivariate comparison of cardiac fluoroscopy, exercise electrocardiography and exercise thallium myocardial perfusion scintigraphy. J Am Coll Cardiol 1984;4:8–16.
47. Melin JA, Wijns W, Vanbutsele RJ *et al.* Alternative diagnostic strategies for coronary artery disease in women: Demonstration of the usefulness and efficiency of probability analysis. Circulation 1985;71:535–42.
48. Robert AR, Melin JA, Detry J-M. Logistic discriminant analysis improves diagnostic accuracy of exercise testing for coronary artery disease in women. Circulation 1991;83:1202–9.
49. Massini M, Picano E, Lattanzi F, Distante A, L'Abbate A. High-dose dipyridamole echocardiography test in women: Correlation with exercise electrocardiography test and coronary arteriography. J Am Coll Cardiol 1988;12:682–5.
50. Sawada SG, Ryan T, Fineberg NS *et al.* Exercise echocardiographic detection of coronary artery disease in women. J Am Coll Cardiol 1989;14:1440–7.
51. Coma-Canella I. Sensitivity and specificity of dobutamine-electrocardiography test to detect multivessel disease after acute myocardial infarction. Eur Heart J 1990;11:249–57.
52. Coma-Canella I. Dobutamine stress test to diagnose the presence and severity of coronary lesions in angina. Eur Heart J 1991;12:1198–204.
53. Sawada SG, Segar DS, Ryan T *et al.* Echocardiographic detection of coronary artery disease during dobutamine infusion. Circulation 1991; 83:1605–14.
54. Cohen JL, Greene TO, Ottenweller J, Binenbaum SZ, Wilchfort SD, Kim CS. Dobutamine digital echocardiography for detecting coronary artery disease. Am J Cardiol 1991;67:1311–8.
55. Marcowitz P, Armstrong WF. Accuracy of dobutamine stress echocardiography in detecting coronary artery disease. Am J Cardiol 1992;69:1269–73.
56. Mairesse G, Marwick T, D'Hondt AM, Wyns W, Melin JA, Detry J-M. How reliable is the dobutamine stress ECG for the diagnosis of coronary disease? A Receiver Operating Curve analysis [abstract]. J Am Coll Cardiol 1993;21:174A.
57. Picano E, Lattanzi F, Masini M, Distante A, L'Abbate A. Usefulness of the dipyridamole-exercise echocardiography test for diagnosis of coronary artery disease. Am J Cardiol 1988;62:67–70.
58. Cohen JL, Greene TO, Alston JR, Wilchford SD, Kim CS. Usefulness of oral dipyridamole digital echocardiography for detecting coronary artery disease. Am J Cardiol 1989;64:385–6.
59. Agati L, Arata L, Peraldo Neja C *et al.* Usefulness of the dipyridamole-Doppler test for diagnosis of coronary artery disease. Am J Cardiol 1990;65:829–34.
60. Marwick T, Willemart B, D'Hondt AM *et al.* Selection of the optimal non-exercise stress for the evaluation of ischemic regional myocardial dysfunction and malperfusion: Comparison of dobutamine and adenosine using echocardiography and Tc-99 m MIBI single photon emission computed tomography. Circulation 1993;87:345–54.
61. Zoghbi WA, Cheirif J, Kleiman NS, Verani MS, Trakhtenbroit A. Diagnosis of ischemic heart disease with adenosine echocardiography. J Am Coll Cardiol 1991;18:1271–98.
62. Picano E. Dipyridamole-echocardiography test: Historical background and physiologic basis. Eur Heart J 1989;10:365–76.

7. Comparison of Stress Echocardiography and Scintigraphic Techniques for the Diagnosis of Coronary Artery Disease

T. MARWICK and J.A. MELIN

Nuclear cardiology techniques may be used to diagnose coronary artery disease by the examination of myocardial function and perfusion at rest and during exercise. Because these methodologies are well established, the efficacy of stress echocardiography as an adjunct (or even, an alternative) warrants particularly careful consideration. However, despite the favorable record of the nuclear techniques, they have disadvantages with respect to cost (of imaging equipment, isotopes and disposables), patient convenience (particularly with thallium imaging) and availability. Nevertheless, the dominant issue in the selection of one or the other technique must be accuracy.

This chapter will attempt to define the place of stress echocardiography in the context of these nuclear imaging techniques. As a number of variables may potentially influence the results of either test, comparisons will focus on studies involving performance of both echocardiographic and nuclear imaging in the same patients. For these comparisons to be valid, we are assuming that the investigators in these studies are equally expert in either technique. Likewise, we assume that practitioners making choices between echocardiography and scintigraphy have equivalent expertise available in each. Indeed, the accessibility of expert performance and interpretation promises to be a paramount issue in the relative clinical diffusion of these approaches.

7.1 Current Status of Scintigraphic Approaches for the Diagnosis of Coronary Artery Disease

7.1.1 *Nuclear Ventriculography*

Ventricular function may be examined before and after exercise using equilibrium nuclear ventriculography (also known as gated blood pool scanning) or radionuclide angiocardiography (also known as first pass nuclear ventriculography). Variable criteria are used to label an exercise ventriculogram as abnormal, but features suggestive of coronary artery disease include; failure to improve ejection fraction in response to stress, failure to attain a specified ejection fraction, and development of new or worsening regional wall motion abnormalities [1–3]. These count-based methods of calculating ejection fractions are particularly favorable in the evaluation of patients with left ven-

T.H. Marwick, Stress Echocardiography, 113–137.

tricles of non-geometric shape, for example, after myocardial infarction. However, the regional function criteria are less reliable, both for technical reasons (see below) and because only endocardial excursion and not thickening data are available. Also, because data are acquired in only one view during exercise (left anterior oblique in gated studies and right anterior oblique and anterior in first-pass studies), the prevalence of regional wall motion abnormalities is significantly lower than that of an abnormal ejection fraction response. When present, however, regional wall motion abnormalities are highly specific for coronary artery disease. The strength of global functional evaluation with nuclear ventriculography and the weakness of regional evaluation contrast with the respective strengths and weaknesses of echocardiography (Chapter 2).

Gated blood pool scanning involves detection of circulating tracer mixed evenly in the blood, with a prolonged period of sampling (5 to 10 minutes of imaging at rest, with 2 to 3 minutes of exercise and post-exercise imaging) to obtain adequate counts. Images are created by the summation of hundreds of cardiac cycles, usually divided into 16 to 24 frames in a cine-loop gated on the R-wave [4,5]. The shortcomings of this technique are inherent in its methodology. The heterogeneity in stroke volumes over many cardiac cycles, together with respiratory and body movement, leads to imperfect definition of the endocardial border, and therefore, of regional systolic function. The duration of exercise imaging means that these data may not necessarily be obtained at peak exercise. Finally, the need to minimize body movement over a long duration of imaging mandates supine (or semi-supine) exercise, which is relatively non-physiologic [6], and during which the patient may be limited by fatigue rather than cardiovascular stress.

The alternative, first pass methodology, is based upon obtaining a relatively high concentration of isotope in the left ventricle over a short time, through injection of the tracer as a rapid bolus [7]. This approach offers good imaging of the right heart chambers, but the bolus may become diluted by the time that it reaches the left side, particularly in patients with heart failure. The main limitations of the gated technique are solved using this approach, which obtains peak exercise images in real time, and may be used with upright exercise. However, images acquired in this fashion are also non-tomographic, so that analysis of left ventricular regional wall motion may still be limited. Moreover, various technical problems may appear with either method, including those due to soft tissue attenuation and labelling of the red blood cells.

The accuracy of stress nuclear ventriculography is dependent upon the criteria employed in its interpretation. In patients with a normal ejection fraction, Jones [7] found criteria of stress-induced regional dysfunction to have high specificity (88%), but low sensitivity (46%). In contrast, global alterations of ejection fraction were more sensitive but less specific. Combining regional and global data in patients with optimal scans gave a sensitivity of 90%, with a specificity of 58%. Prospective application of the criteria previously developed in 486 patients to a new series of 221 similar patients identified a sensitivity of 87% and a specificity of 54% [8]. The lack of augmentation of ejection fraction from rest to exercise has been used to label a radionuclide angiogram as abnormal, but as the change in ejection fraction from rest to exercise is a complex response influenced by many variables [9,10], and the peak exercise ejection fraction has been found to be a better parameter for the detection of coronary disease [11]. The observation that absolute ejection fraction provided more diagnostic information than change in ejection fraction has been confirmed by a large patient group assembled from several centers [12]. Finally, the low specificity of the global ejection fraction parameter can be explained by different factors such as patient selection considerations [13,14], physiologic factors [15,16] affecting ventricular function during exercise (such to age and gender), and the obligate use of symptomatic patients with normal coronary arteriograms to define specificity.

7.1.2 *Myocardial Perfusion Imaging*

The basic principle of scintigraphic perfusion imaging is that myocardial tracer activity reflects perfusion and viability, because selected intravenously-administered radioisotopes concentrate in the myocardium [17]. Within regions of infarction, the absence of viable cells to concentrate the tracer prevents its uptake in the resting state. A similar picture may be obtained with viable tissue subtended by an obstructed artery, although in this situation, it is the absence of tracer delivery rather than the absence of tracer uptake which is the cause of the perfusion defect. The majority of injected Tl-201 is taken up in non-cardiac sites immediately after injection – because of its long half-life, Tl-201 continues to be delivered to the myocardium from these sites, and continues to be concentrated by viable myocytes in regions supplied by occluded vessels. Such viable regions therefore show redistribution on late (24 hour) images, or following thallium reinjection [18,19].

Arteries with significant ($\geqslant$ 50% diameter) stenoses do not usually cause abnormal perfusion at rest [20], but do limit the ability to increase coronary flow by vasodilation (induced by either exercise or dipyridamole). Non-homogeneity of coronary vasodilation (analogous to measurement of coronary flow reserve) in different territories thereby identifies coronary stenoses, provided that this non-uniformity was not present at rest. It is important to note that for perfusion scintigraphy, stress techniques are based on causing coronary vasodilation rather than necessarily inducing ischemia in a functional or metabolic sense. Pre-existing coronary vasodilation induced by anti-anginal therapy, and limitation of the vasodilator response to exercise by limiting heart rate response are therefore potential problems. Submaximal augmentation of coronary flow (caused by either submaximal exercise or dipyridamole unresponsiveness), may not permit detection of less severe stenoses, contributing to lower sensitivity [21].

Conventional planar imaging (performed in 3 views) is limited by relatively poor spatial resolution, and ambiguity about the quantity of malperfused tissue. Tomographic imaging (SPECT) has improved Tl sensitivity from around 85% with planar techniques to around 95% [22], improved the localization of defects [23] and assessment of defect size, and facilitated a global evaluation of the heart (using polar map displays). However, the performance of SPECT takes longer, costs more, is technically demanding, and has problems with specificity [24].

The greatest problems with Tl-201 imaging reflect the physical properties of this compound [25]. Thallium produces low energy photons (69–83 KeV) which are readily attenuated by soft tissue (causing false positive defects and suboptimal imaging of deep structures), and are prone to scatter (causing poor spatial resolution). Counts are also limited by radiation dosimetry. Some of these disadvantages have been ameliorated by use of the isonitriles as bloodflow tracers. This group of synthetic, Tc-99 m-tagged compounds, such as sestamethoxybutylisonitrile (MIBI) has advantages over Tl-201 with respect to higher energy emissions, more favorable radiation dosimetry, generation on-site, and availability of a true resting scan. Despite these theoretical advantages, however, the accuracy of myocardial perfusion imaging using the isonitriles is comparable to that of Tl-201, rather than being significantly better [26]. Moreover, a problem common to both Tl-201 and MIBI-SPECT studies is variable attenuation caused by varying distance of myocardial regions from the collimator and variable tissue thickness interposed between the myocardium and the collimator. These attenuation patterns are frequently the source of false positive studies, and various algorithms are being developed which are aimed at correcting for attenuation and scatter. Alternatively, because of its high count rates, planar or SPECT MIBI images may be acquired with cardiac gating to assess wall thickening in addition to myocardial perfusion. The review of gated MIBI data should offer an additional quality control method for identifying SPECT imaging attenuation artifacts.

Positron emission tomography (PET) has advantages over conventional scintigraphic methods in relation to attenuation correction, higher energy emissions (which limit problems with attenuation artifacts and improve imaging of the inferoposterior aspect of heart), availability of a true resting scan, and improved contrast and spatial resolution. These theoretical benefits have been translated into greater levels of accuracy [27]. One study in 203 patients performed with near simultaneous injection of Rb-82 and Tl-201, reported similar specificities of 78% and 80% for PET and SPECT. The sensitivity was 93% for PET compared with only 76% for SPECT [28]. A second study, comparing exercise or dipyridamole stress Tl-201 SPECT to Rb-82 dipyridamole stress PET in 81 patients, reported similar sensitivities for both approaches but a significant gain in specificity with PET from 53% to 88% [29]. However, PET remains too expensive to be applicable as a clinical tool in other than the largest of referral centers.

7.2 Accuracy of Stress Echocardiography versus Stress Nuclear Ventriculography

On theoretical grounds, echocardiography and gated nuclear ventriculography examine different aspects of imaging the left ventricle, as discussed above. The strength of nuclear ventriculography is in the accurate assessment of global function, while the evaluation of regional function is the strength of echocardiography. Despite these considerations, the ability to appreciate changes in global left ventricular performance with echocardiography and gated nuclear ventriculography are comparable [30], as are evaluations of regional function with echocardiography and first pass ventriculography [31]. However, in contrast to the nuclear ventriculography methodologies, echocardiography can offer imaging of multiple planes at peak stress, has good spatial resolution and edge detection (hence reliably examines regional wall motion), and may be used to analyze myocardial thickening. Because nonischemic myocardium develops hyperkinesis to compensate for ischemic dysfunction in other areas, disturbances of global left ventricular function usually reflect extensive ischemia, while milder ischemia may produce no alteration in the ejection fraction. In contrast, the compensatory response of normal myocardium enhances the appreciation of regional wall motion disturbances using stress echocardiography.

These theoretical considerations are supported by limited data obtained by direct comparison of exercise echocardiography and exercise nuclear ventriculography [32–34]. In these studies, global and/or regional criteria were used for the assessment of nuclear scans (Table 7.1). Comparison of the sensitivities in only 70 patients show that stress echocardiography is more sensitive than nuclear ventriculography for the identification of myocardial ischemia. Comparison of the specificities of stress echocardiography and nuclear ventriculography has been reported in only 30 patients. In studies using global functional criteria, the specificity of nuclear ventriculography may be compromised by false positives caused by exercise-induced impairment of the ejection fraction in patients with hypertrophic and valvular heart diseases [35]. In this group, the specificity of nuclear ventriculography (an ejection fraction-based test) might be expected to be inferior to that of stress echocardiography (whose interpretation does not usually include ejection fraction analysis). While the available reports suggest stress echocardiography and nuclear ventriculography are equivalent, studies in larger, unselected groups may confirm the superiority of echocardiography, reflecting its strength in the evaluation of regional function.

In conclusion, comparisons of stress echocardiography and stress nuclear ventriculography show them to have similar accuracy, with echocardiography having some benefit in terms of sensitivity. Although technically more demanding, echocardiography also has the benefits of lower cost, providing other anatomic information (regarding the valves and pericardium), and is more tomographic.

Table 7.1. Comparison of sensitivity and specificity of exercise stress echocardiography and the exerci

Author	Ref	n	Nuclear methodology	LV function criteria	Sensitivity – echo	Sensitivity – nuclear
Limacher	32	24	Supine MUGA	EF reduction or WM abn	92% (n = 24)	71% (n = 24)
Visser	33	35	Supine MUGA	Regional WM abn	86% (n = 22)	91% (n = 22)
Crawford	34	18	Upright MUGA	EF reduction	89% (n = 18)	77% (n = 18)

Echo = exercise echocardiogram, EF = ejection fraction, LV = left ventricular, MI = myocardi number, WM = wall motion.

7.3 Accuracy of Stress Echocardiography versus Perfusion Scintigraphy

Myocardial perfusion scintigraphy is currently the most widely used imaging technique for the non-invasive diagnosis of coronary artery disease. The advantages and disadvantages of each test are summarized in Table 7.2. Thallium imaging is relatively automated, but has the disadvantages of being costly, time-consuming for the patient (because of redistribution imaging), involves radiation exposure, and may have problems with specificity due to artifacts. Stress echocardiography does not share these technical problems and can offer real-time imaging of the heart (possibly enhancing safety and enabling visualization of the time-course of ischemia), but is technically more difficult. The influence of these considerations on the relative accuracy of each test can only be addressed by direct comparison of the tests in the same patient population.

On theoretical grounds, perfusion scintigraphy identifies the presence of coronary disease on the basis of stress-induced perfusion heterogeneity – which may not necessarily parallel the presence of myocardial ischemia, especially in the setting of vasodilator stress [36]. Thus a stenosis may be identified by perfusion scintigraphy when coronary flow increases after vasodilation by only two-fold, compared with four-fold in a normal zone, even though the oxygen requirements of the stenosed zone are adequate to prevent ischemia in a metabolic or functional sense. This difference between the techniques also causes drug therapy (which prevents the development of ischemia) to influence the results of echocardiography [37], while it does not influence the results of perfusion scintigraphy [38], because the latter examines coronary supply (which is little influenced by drug therapy). This perfusion-function discrepancy is less liable to occur with exercise stress, as the vasodilator effect of stress more closely parallels myocardial metabolic requirements. For these reasons, studies comparing perfusion scintigraphy and stress echocardiography using exercise (or dobutamine) and vasodilator stress will be considered separately.

nuclear ventriculography for the detection of coronary artery disease.

Specificity – echo	Specificity – nuclear	Comments	Detection SVD – echo	Detection SVD – ECG
88% (n = 17)	82% (n = 17)	MI pts included	64% (n = 11)	64% (n = 11)
92% (n = 13)	100% (n = 13)	MI pts excluded	60% (n = 5)	60% (n = 5)
–	–	MI pts included	NS	NS

infarction, MUGA = gated nuclear ventriculogram, pts = patients, ref = reference

Table 7.2. Comparison of advantages and disadvantages of stress echocardiography and myocardial perfusion imaging.

	Stress echocardiography	Stress thallium imaging
Equipment	Low cost Portable	Expensive Laboratory-based
Personnel	"Learning curve" for acquisition/reading	Relatively automated License necessary
Imaging	No radiation Rapid, instant results Tomographic Imaging during exercise, at peak & post	Small radiation exposure Long protocols Planar vs SPECT "Snapshot" at peak exercise
Reporting	Regional function/thickening Usually qualitative Global function available (EF,ESV)	Regional flow heterogeneity Quantitation well accepted Global indices available (TID, lung-heart ratio)
Benefits	Identifies other sources of chest pain	Viability data available
Problems	Technically difficult studies Interpretation of infarct zones	Artifacts LV hypertrophy, Left bundle branch block

7.3.1 *Exercise (or Dobutamine) Stress Echocardiography and Perfusion Scintigraphy*

The sensitivity and specificity values reported in studies involving exercise (or dobutamine) stress echocardiography and stress perfusion scintigraphy in the same patients are summarized in Table 7.3 [39–44]. These studies have been selected because of the direct comparison of both tests with angiographic data as the reference standard. Other studies have involved cath-

Table 7.3. Comparison of sensitivity and specificity of echocardiography and myocardial

Author	Ref	n	Significant stenosis	Stress methodology	Nuclear methodology	Sensitivity – echo
Maurer	39	36	>50%	Treadmill	Planar Tl	83% (n = 23)
Galanti	40	53	>70%	Upright bike	Planar Tl	93% (n = 27)
Pozzoli	41	75	>50%	Upright bike	SPECT-MIBI	71% (n = 49)
Salustri	42	44	>50%	Upright bike	SPECT-MIBI/Tl	86% (n = 30)
Quinones	43	112	>50%	Treadmill	SPECT-Tl	74% (n = 86)
Marwick	44	217	>50%	Db 40 mcg/kg/min	SPECT-MIBI	72% (n = 142)
Perin	47	25	>50%	Dipy 0.56 mg/kg	SPECT-Tl	58% (n = 19)
Simonetti	48	35	>75%	Dipy 0.84 mg/kg	Planar Tl	86% (n = 22)
Parodi	49	79	>50%	Dipy 0.84 mg/kg	SPECT-MIBI	73% (n = 60)
Marwick	50	97	>50%	Ad 0.18 mg/kg/min	SPECT-MIBI	58% (n = 59)

AD = adenosine, CAD = coronary artery disease, Dipy = dipyridamole, Echo = exercise Tl = thallium, WMA = wall motion abnormality.

eterization in subgroups of patients, and will not be discussed because of the absence of a reference standard for all patients.

The sensitivities of both tests for the identification of coronary artery disease are comparable. The theoretical superiority of perfusion imaging for the detection of mild ischemia (evident as flow heterogeneity) was evidenced in practice in one study [41] which showed a benefit for perfusion imaging in the setting of single vessel coronary artery disease. The confirmation of this in only a single study may reflect the inclusion of mild (50–70% stenoses) in the coronary disease subgroup, as well as the appropriate exclusion of patients with resting ECG abnormalities.

The values for specificity recorded in these studies are also comparable between echocardiography and perfusion scintigraphy, with most series showing a small benefit for echocardiography. These data are also consistent with previous data which indicate that the high sensitivity of myocardial perfusion imaging with SPECT is at the cost of a sacrifice in specificity [24]. Concordance rates between scintigraphy and echocardiography for the presence or absence of disease range from 80 to 90% in most studies.

The results of direct comparisons of exercise and dobutamine stress echocardiography and perfusion scintigraphy presented in this chapter suggest that the two techniques offer comparable levels of accuracy in the diagnosis of coronary artery disease. This equivalence is contrary to the results expected from the "ischemic cascade" model (Chapter 1) – as the development of a perfusion disturbance initiates ischemia, perfusion imaging might be expected to be more sensitive than wall motion imaging for the detection of ischemia. However, the relative performance of each modality is determined not only by the underlying physiology, but also by its imaging characteristics. Various strengths of the echocardiographic technique may compensate for the development of dysfunction after perfusion abnormalities, including improved spatial resolution, and the ability to categorize wall motion independently in each segment (contrasting with the relative flow comparisons used

perfusion imaging after various stressors for the detection of coronary artery disease.

Sensitivity – nuclear	Sens-SVD – echo	Sens-SVD – nuclear	Specificity – echo	Specificity – nuclear	Exclusions
74% (n = 23)	50% (n = 6)	–	92% (n = 13)	92% (n = 13)	MI
100% (n = 27)	93% (n = 14)	100% (n = 14)	96% (n = 26)	92% (n = 26)	MI, resting WMA
84% (n = 49)	60% (n = 33)	82% (n = 33)	96% (n = 26)	88% (n = 26)	Abn resting ECG
83% (n = 30)	86% (n = 30)	83% (n = 30)	85% (n = 14)	64% (n = 14)	Multivessel CAD
76% (n = 86)	58% (n = 41)	61% (n = 41)	88% (n = 26)	81% (n = 26)	-
76% (n = 142)	66% (n = 68)	74% (n = 68)	83% (n = 75)	67% (n = 75)	MI
95% (n = 19)	-	-	100% (n = 6)	50% (n = 6)	-
91% (n = 22)	-	-	92% (n = 13)	100% (n = 13)	MI
77% (n = 60)	-	-	84% (n = 19)	84% (n = 19)	MI
86% (n = 59)	52% (n = 31)	81% (n = 31)	87% (n = 38)	71% (n = 38)	MI

echocardiogram, MI = myocardial infarction, ref = reference number, SVD = single vessel disease,

in myocardial perfusion imaging). Some ischemic regions may even be identified by echocardiography rather than scintigraphy – for example, abnormal wall motion due to subendocardial ischemia may be evident before malperfusion is extensive enough (horizontally and vertically) to be apparent at perfusion scintigraphy.

7.3.2 *Vasodilator Stress Echocardiography versus Perfusion Scintigraphy*

As discussed in Chapter 5, the coronary steal induced by dipyridamole is rarely responsible for extensive ischemia of the variety needed to cause global ventricular dysfunction. Thus, despite early studies showing concordance between stroke volume changes and perfusion defects at thallium imaging [45], subsequent studies have shown no reliable correlation between the two [46,47]. Studies comparing the regional functional responses of vasodilator stress echocardiography and perfusion imaging, with catheterization data are summarized in Table 7.3 [47–50]. Perfusion heterogeneity may be induced at standard vasodilator doses, but steal phenomena (hence metabolic or functional evidence of ischemia) are generally not [36]. Hence, studies report that perfusion imaging is more sensitive than echocardiography during standard doses of dipyridamole (0.56 mg/kg). Using a high-dose protocol, echocardiography during dipyridamole [47] or adenosine [50] stress was less sensitive than perfusion scintigraphy. This finding was less prominent in those with multivessel disease, though scintigraphy was more sensitive in both single and multivessel disease groups (Figure 7.1). This superiority of scintigraphy is not apparent with dobutamine or exercise stress (see below).

The comparison of echocardiography and perfusion scintigraphy using vasodilator stress places the former at an intrinsic disadvantage, as this form of stress is not optimal for echocardiography, while it is for scintigraphy (see Chapter 5). Comparisons have also been made between the techniques using the best stress for each – exercise [51,52] or dobutamine [50] for echocardio-

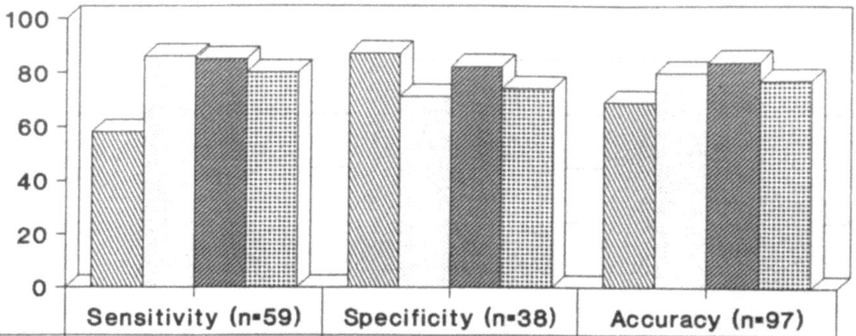

	Sensitivity (n=59)	Specificity (n=38)	Accuracy (n=97)
AdEcho	58	87	69
AdMIBI	86	71	80
DbEcho	85	82	84
DbMIBI	80	74	77

AdEcho AdMIBI DbEcho DbMIBI

Figure 7.1. Comparison of accuracies of adenosine stress echocardiography and MIBI-SPECT and dobutamine stress echocardiography and MIBI-SPECT in unselected patients undergoing coronary angiography [50]. Reproduced with permission of the American Heart Association.

graphy, and a vasodilator for scintigraphy. Under such circumstances, the sensitivities of the tests are comparable, though the specificity of echocardiography exceeds that of scintigraphy.

7.3.3 *Combination of Stress Echocardiography and Perfusion Scintigraphy*

The roles of functional and perfusion imaging might potentially be complementary in the diagnosis of coronary disease, with scintigraphy sometimes showing greater accuracy because of the earlier development of perfusion heterogeneity in the ischemic cascade, and echocardiography showing greater accuracy in other instances, as described previously. We therefore investigated the results of combining perfusion imaging with dobutamine stress echocardiograms in all or some of a study group of 217 patients [44]. The sensitivity, specificity and accuracy of these combined approaches is portrayed in Figure 7.2. The first combination is to employ both tests in all patients – this maximizes the sensitivity (89%), but compromises the specificity by combining the false positives of each methodology (specificity 52%). This option is therefore not feasible on grounds of cost or results. As the specificity of echocardiography is high, the next alternative is to combine the tests only in patients in whom echocardiography is negative. This option offers the same results as the first combination, with the performance of

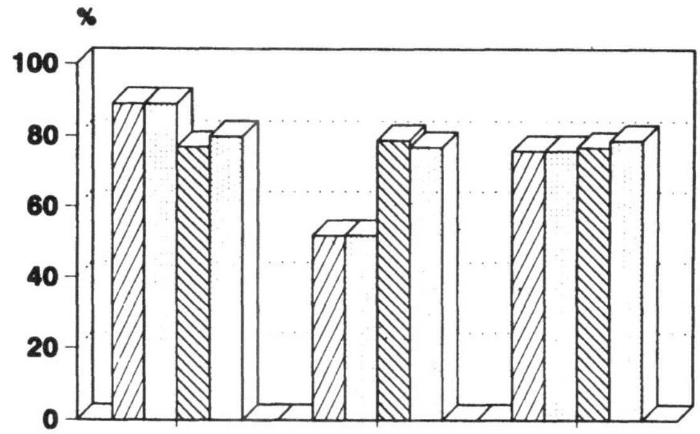

DbE combined with MIBI-SPECT in;	Sensitivity	Specificity	Accuracy
All patients	89	52	76
Negative DbE	89	52	76
Submax DbE(ex LVH,LBB)	77	79	77
Neg submax DbE	80	77	79

All patients Negative DbE Submax DbE(ex LVH,LBB) Neg submax DbE

Figure 7.2. Sensitivity, specificity and accuracy of combinations of dobutamine echocardiography (DbE) and perfusion imaging (using MIBI-SPECT) for the diagnosis of coronary artery disease in unselected patients [44]. The four combinations comprise use of MIBI-SPECT in all patients, and restriction to those with a negative DbE, a submaximal DbE (except patients with LBBB and LVH, in whom DbE may avoid false positive perfusion results), and submaximal DbE only in those with negative scans. Reproduced with permission of the Journal of the American College of Cardiology.

fewer scintigrams (in 47%), but to be useful clinically, requires on-line interpretation.

The third and fourth alternatives focus on the use of echocardiography as a preliminary test, combining with Tc99 m MIBI perfusion scintigraphy in those with submaximal tests (patients on beta-blocking drugs, or in whom the maximal dobutamine dose is not attained). If this approach is combined with the avoidance of perfusion imaging in any patient with left ventricular hypertrophy and left bundle branch block (the major sources of false positive perfusion imaging results – see below), a further reduction of the number of scintigrams can be achieved (to 29%), and gives a high sensitivity without compromising specificity to the same extent. Additional reduction in the number of scintigrams (to 14%) with comparable enhancement of sensitivity can be achieved by the use of scintigraphy only in those with a negative submaximal dobutamine echocardiogram may further limit the number of required studies (n = 30), while at the same time increasing the sensitivity of dobutamine echocardiography alone. The latter two alternatives represent the most efficient combinations of scintigraphy with dobutamine echocardiography.

7.4 Identification of Myocardial Ischemia or Infarction Using Stress Echocardiography or Scintigraphy

While these data on sensitivity and specificity are of use in comparing the tests in the diagnosis of coronary disease, this is not always the question clinically. In patients after myocardial infarction, this analysis is somewhat limited, as it does not discriminate between the diagnoses of scar and ischemia. In order to elucidate this point, a comparison of the type of abnormality is required on a regional basis.

While the concordance between echocardiography and perfusion scintigraphy for the presence or absence of coronary artery disease is usually 80 to 90%, the agreement between the tests is usually about 10% less with respect to the identification of normal, ischemic or infarcted myocardium [51,52]. This heterogeneity occurs because the interpretation of ischemia or infarction with both perfusion scintigraphy and echocardiography is ambiguous. A "fixed" thallium perfusion defect at 4 hours may indicate severe ischemia rather than scar [53], and combinations of ischemia by echocardiography and "scar" by perfusion scintigraphy are often not associated with a history of prior infarction or Q waves in the corresponding segment [52]. These features suggest that the echocardiographic diagnosis is correct – but definitive proof awaits the comparison with a "gold standard" of viability (myocardial metabolic imaging or follow-up after revascularization). Likewise, resting akinesia may be due to tethering of normal myocardium due to adjacent scar [54], stunning or hibernation (see Chapter 10), and not only infarction (Figure 7.3). Moreover, the deterioration of function in ischemic myocardium may involve a change from abnormal to more abnormal – which is more difficult to identify than alterations from normal function. Patients with resting dysfunction therefore have more discordant results than those with normal function, and thallium imaging may be more reliable than stress echocardiography for visualization of the infarct- and peri-infarct zones after myocardial infarction [43]. Again, however, the final clarification of this matter must await interpretation of these mismatched diagnoses in the light of an independent reference standard other than angiography, which merely identifies the presence of coronary disease rather than its effects upon the myocardium.

7.5 Assessment of Disease Localization and Extent Using Stress Echocardiography and Scintigraphy

The posterior regions of the heart may not be reliably assessed with perfusion scintigraphy, due to problems of photon attenuation. This problem appears to be less prominent with echocardiography, which more readily detects the sequelae of coronary stenoses involving the inferior wall [43], although other data conflict with this interpretation [42]. On the other hand, echocardiographic interpretation of wall motion abnormalities in the circumflex territory

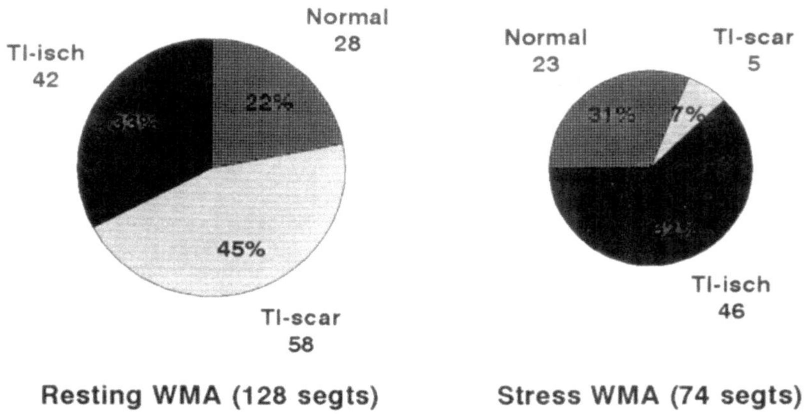

Figure 7.3. Tl-SPECT findings among patients with resting and stress-induced left ventricular dysfunction. Segments with resting wall motion abnormalities show more discordant results at scintigraphy than those with stress-induced wall motion abnormalities. Modified from Quinones [43].

may be compromised by poor endocardial definition in the apical 4–chamber views of the lateral wall. A corresponding benefit of scintigraphy over echocardiography in these segments has been suggested by Pozzoli [41]. However, in larger numbers of patients, regional analyses failed to show significant benefits of either test for the detection of either anterior or posterior territory disease.

We have compared the ability of echocardiography and perfusion scintigraphy to predict coronary disease extent in a series of over 200 patients, studied by both techniques [44]. Using a standard algorithm to reflect the perfusion territories of the coronary arteries, dobutamine stress echocardiography identified 18% of the 74 patients with multivessel coronary disease as having functional abnormalities in >1 coronary territory, compared with scintigrams showing a multivessel pattern in 34% (p = NS). On the other hand, echocardiography was more specific for multivessel disease, which it predicted incorrectly in 9% of patients having single vessel disease, compared with 19% falsely predicted by perfusion imaging. The ability of each test to recognize multivessel disease was also analysed by correlating the echocardiographic or perfusion extent score (calculated from the number of segments demonstrating abnormal regional function or perfusion, expressed as a percentage of the visible segments – usually 16), with an angiographic score of disease extent (modified from the Gensini score). The echocardiographic and scintigraphic correlation with the angiographic score corresponded to a similar degree, with respective R values of 0.45 and 0.35. These data indicated that functional and perfusion indices of coronary disease extent are comparable, and have similar overall accuracy in predicting (but underestimating) multivessel disease.

7.6 Situations of Intrinsic Benefit for Stress Echocardiography versus Scintigraphy

While some artifacts are readily recognized as such at perfusion scintigraphy [55], there are some patient subgroups who continue to generate disproportionate numbers of false positive scintigrams – in particular, women, patients with left bundle branch block and those with left ventricular hypertrophy. The accuracy of stress echocardiography has been established in women (see Chapter 6), although no series attending to the direct comparison with perfusion scintigraphy in women has thus far been reported.

Patients with left bundle branch block (as well as paced rhythms) typically demonstrate false positive perfusion defects in the territory of the left anterior descending coronary artery [56–58]. The cause of false positive perfusion imaging in the presence of left bundle branch block remains uncertain. The most likely explanation is that asynchronous activation of the septum may cause this to contract during part of diastole, which is the time that coronary perfusion is maximal. A perfusion defect may therefore arise at rest, or (more commonly) be induced by exercise, when diastole is further shortened. Thus, the use of a vasodilator stress (which does not normally induce significant tachycardia) may avoid this problem [57]. Other authors have suggested that patients with known left bundle branch block should only be identified as showing ischemia if the apex is involved in the perfusion defect [58].

Left bundle branch block also interferes with the interpretation of stress nuclear ventriculography, both due to regional and global functional changes [59,60]. The ability of echocardiography to examine left ventricular thickening, as well as its ability to interrogate other left anterior descending territory regions than the septum, may circumvent these problems. Reports involving a few patients with left bundle branch block appear to show that stress echocardiography (Figure 7.4) does not share the false positive results of perfusion imaging [44].

As discussed in Chapter 6, coronary artery disease and left ventricular hypertrophy frequently co-exist. Not only is ECG stress testing problematic – perfusion scintigraphy in these patients shows a suboptimal accuracy [61]. False positive resting [62] or stress-induced defects [63] reflect both imaging considerations and the physiologic sequelae of left ventricular hypertrophy (heterogeneity of regional flow reserve). False negative perfusion scintigraphy may also arise due to the effects of hypertrophy on the coronary microcir-

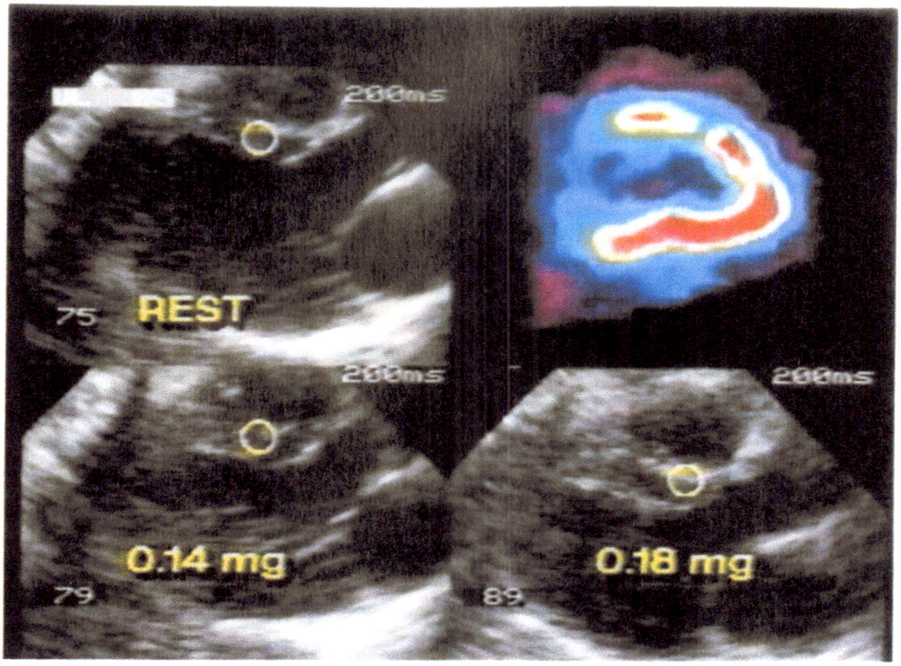

Figure 7.4. Results of adenosine stress echocardiography and MIBI-SPECT in a patient with left bundle branch block and normal coronary arteries. Scintigraphy (upper right) reveals an anteroseptal perfusion defect. Systolic images at rest and during adenosine stress demonstrate normal myocardial thickening at the same site (circled).

culation. The development of left ventricular hypertrophy may be associated with inadequate growth of the coronary vasculature, as well as alterations of vascular geometry [64]. This is compensated by augmentation of resting myocardial bloodflow [65], although despite this, resting regional flow per gram of tissue may be diminished [66]. As resting flow is increased and maximal flow remains the same or is reduced [66–68], flow reserve is reduced even in the absence of coronary disease [69]. The augmentation of tracer uptake into normal tissue after vasodilator stress is reduced, so the difference between a normal area and one supplied by a stenosed artery may be less apparent, analogous to the situation of submaximal exercise. These phenomena have been shown to reduce the sensitivity of dipyridamole stress PET perfusion imaging [70], where the sensitivity was 55% in 20 patients with left ventricular hypertrophy, and 85% in 34 patients with normal left ventricular mass ($p = 0.03$), despite the groups being matched for other clinical, treatment and angiographic variables which influence sensitivity (Figure 7.5).

The lack of any compromise in the accuracy of exercise echocardiography due to hypertrophy has been discussed in Chapter 6 – indeed, the absence

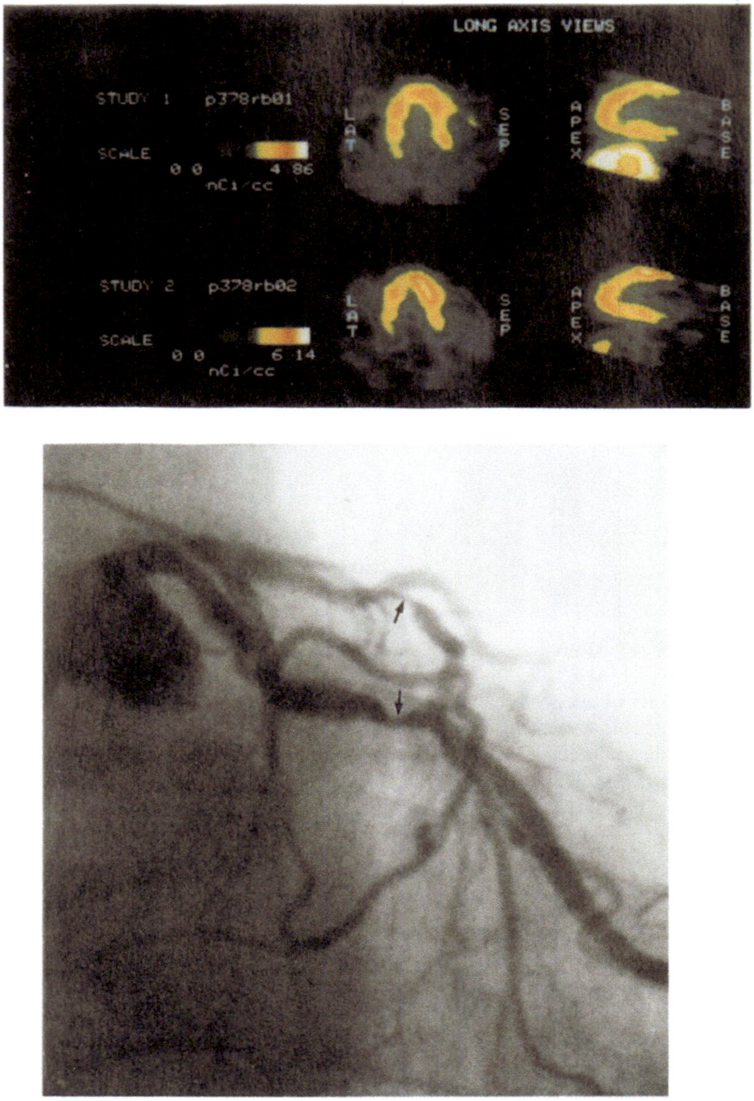

Figure 7.5. False negative PET perfusion scintigraphy with LV hypertrophy. Perfusion is homogeneous at rest ("rb01") and stress ("rb02") despite two-vessel coronary disease (bottom).

of coronary disease in those with left ventricular hypertrophy was more reliably defined than in those with normal left ventricular mass. These findings have been confirmed in a direct comparison with myocardial perfusion scintigraphy (Figure 7.6); dobutamine stress echocardiography was more

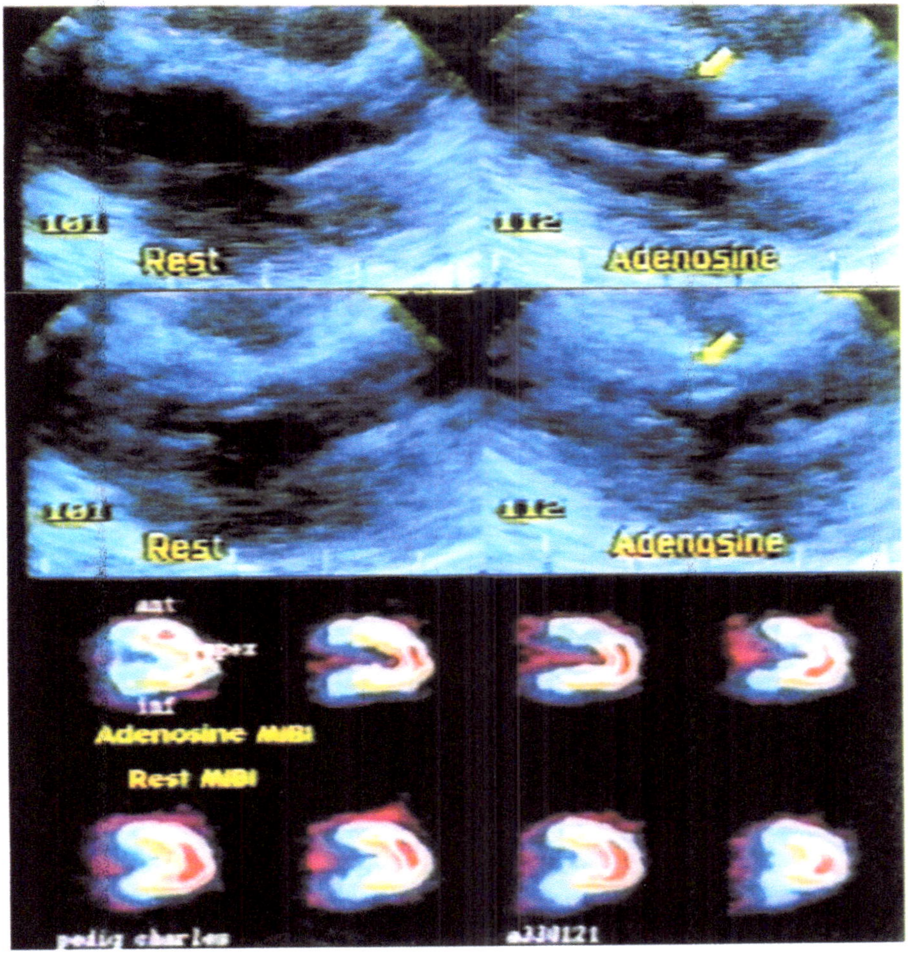

Figure 7.6. Adenosine stress echocardiography and MIBI-SPECT in a patient with normal coronary arteries and left ventricular hypertrophy. The hypertrophied septum (arrows) thickens normally between diastole (top) and systole, at rest and during dipyridamole stress. Scintigraphy reveals a false positive perfusion defect after adenosine, with a partial defect at rest.

specific than perfusion scintigraphy in 75 patients with $< 50\%$ stenoses particularly in the 17 patients with left ventricular hypertrophy but without coronary disease, where the specificity of echocardiography (94%) was significantly greater than that of scintigraphy (59%, $p = 0.02$). Indeed, division of the specificity group into subgroups with and without left ventricular hypertrophy or left bundle branch block (Figure 7.7), showed that the lower overall specificity of dobutamine scintigraphy was chiefly attributable to the false positives associated with the former group [44].

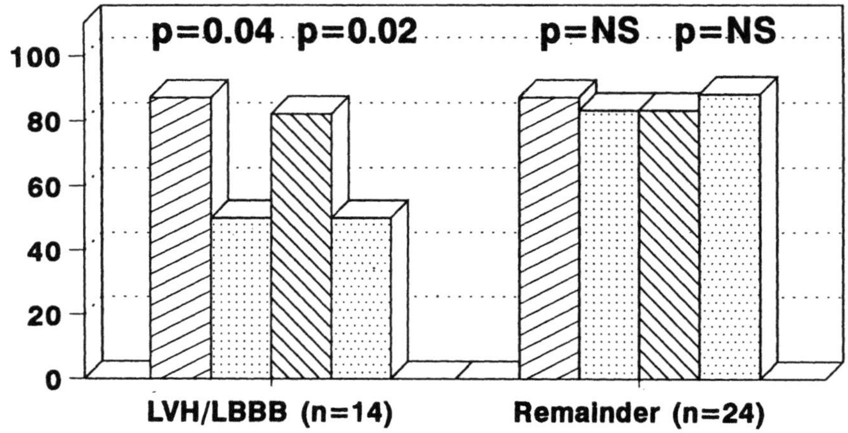

	LVH/LBBB (n=14)	Remainder (n=24)
AdEcho	87	87
AdMIBI	50	83
DbEcho	82	83
DbMIBI	50	88

AdEcho AdMIBI DbEcho DbMIBI

Pts without MI

Figure 7.7. Specificity of stress echocardiography (echo) and perfusion scintigraphy (MIBI-SPECT) in patients with left ventricular hypertrophy (LVH) or left bundle branch block (LBBB), compared with the specificities in patients without these abnormalities. Reproduced with permission of the American Heart Association.

7.7 Stress Echocardiography versus Scintigraphy – A Bayesian Approach

While values for sensitivity and specificity have a useful role in comparing tests, the use of these investigations in diagnostic practice is to assist in the clinical recognition of coronary disease. In this sense, tests are used to reclassify the initial clinical impression of the probability of coronary disease into high-, low- and intermediate-risk subgroups. According to Bayes' theorem, the likelihood of a positive test result is determined by the probability of disease in the patient studied, as well as the accuracy of the test. A comparison of tests using probability analysis permits examination of their performance in groups with various pre-test likelihoods of disease. We performed this analysis in 217 patients studied with dobutamine echocardiography and MIBI-SPECT [44]. The pre-test disease probability, and the post-test probability (derived from the pre-test probability and the odds ratios calculated from values for sensitivity and specificity) were estimated in all patients. The population was grouped into those at high- (>80%), intermediate- (20–80%) and low-probability (<20%) of disease, before and after the performance of each test, and the ability of each test to re-stratify patients was analyzed (Figure 7.8). By application of Bayes' theorem, echocardiography defined 139 patients (64%) as being in the high- or low-probability groups, compared with 110 (51%) using scintigraphy ($p = 0.005$), thus leaving more patients in the intermediate-probability group after scintigraphy. The accuracy of predicting coronary disease in the high probability group, and the absence of disease in the low-probability group was similar for echocardiography (120/139, 86%) and scintigraphy (99/110, 90%).

7.8 Conclusion – Selection of Stress Echocardiography or Perfusion Scintigraphy for the Diagnosis of Coronary Disease

As discussed in the conclusion to Chapter 6, there is currently no rationale for the uniform substitution of the exercise ECG with stress echocardiography. The indications for perfusion scintigraphy and stress echocardiography are therefore similar;

1. Diagnosis of coronary artery disease in patients unsuitable for routine exercise testing or in patients with an intermediate risk of disease,
2. Assessment of the physiologic significance of known coronary stenosis,
3. Assessment of prognosis, as determined from the quantity of infarcted tissue, and the amount of ischemic tissue,
4. Follow-up after intervention.

This chapter has concentrated on the comparison of perfusion imaging and stress echocardiography for diagnostic purposes; comparisons related to other aspects will be discussed briefly in other chapters.

Some features of stress testing with echocardiography and perfusion scintigraphy are comparable – for example, their sensitivity for the diagnosis of coronary disease, and their ability to identify the site (and to a lesser degree, the extent) of disease. Both techniques also have their strong and weak points. Echocardiography requires less equipment (and costs less) than scintigraphy. However, at the present state of development, stress echocardiography is highly operator dependent. Irrespective of other considerations if there is no local expertise in stress echocardiography, its use in preference to the nuclear techniques is highly inappropriate. However, once this condition is fulfilled, we believe that the selection of one or other test should be tailored to clinical circumstances rather than as a uniform decision. To this end, we propose the following guidelines.

Perfusion imaging is more useful in;

1. Post-infarction patients. Thallium scintigraphy is probably more able to identify combinations of ischemia and infarction [43], is accurate for the detection of viable myocardium (although dobutamine echocardiography

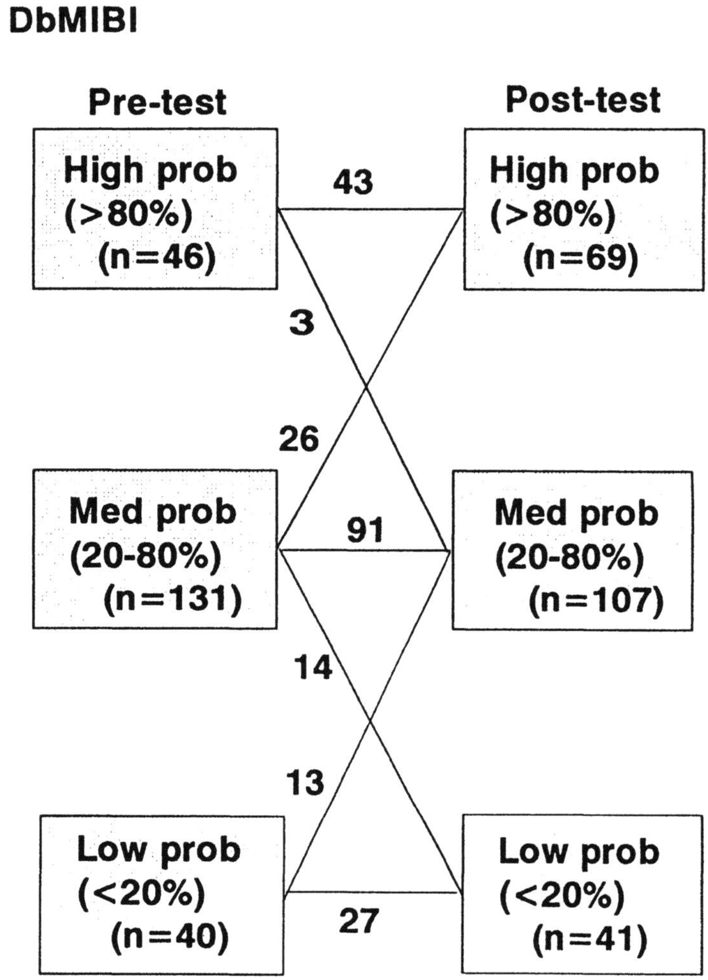

Figure 7.8. A Bayesian approach to the comparison of dobutamine stress echocardiography (right) and MIBI-SPECT (left). Patients are classified before and after the test into low-, intermediate- and high-probability of coronary disease, and the ability of each test to accurately re-classify them is compared (see text).

is promising in this respect), and lacks the problem of peri-infarct tethering seen with echocardiography,

2. Patients requiring vasodilator stress (those unable to exercise and also unable to undergo dobutamine testing). Only perfusion imaging is recommended for diagnostic purposes, as vasodilator echocardiography is insensitive, particularly for single vessel disease.
3. Patients with poor echocardiographic windows (though these individuals

are difficult to predict without performing resting imaging, and the window may paradoxically improve with post-exercise hyperventilation).

Echocardiography is more useful in;

1. Those with left ventricular hypertrophy and left bundle branch block. Stress echocardiography appears to be more specific than perfusion scintigraphy in these situations (though these data await confirmation).
2. Patients in whom safety is a major concern (potentially unstable or severely ischemic). Using echocardiography, ischemia may be observed "on-line" and the appropriate action taken.
3. Studies being performed to assess the adequacy of therapy – as echocardiography visualizes ischemia rather than perfusion heterogeneity, and provides an additional index of disease severity by measuring the ischemia-free stress time.
4. Patients with a suspicion of significant valvular, myocardial or pericardial components to their presentation.

The combination of echocardiography and scintigraphy cannot be recommended because of cost constraints. However, as particular features of stress testing have been identified in which echocardiography is inaccurate (submaximal exercise, submaximal pharmacologic protocols), it may be useful to perform stress echocardiography as the procedure of choice, with the ability to inject Tc-99M MIBI in such circumstances. This option has only become feasible with the availability of MIBI, which does not undergo redistribution. This strategy is accurate as well as cost-efficient.

In a majority of stable patients without a history of infarction, left ventricular hypertrophy or left bundle branch block, who are able to exercise or undergo dobutamine stress, these guidelines leave the decision of echocardiography versus scintigraphy unresolved. Further large studies are needed to elucidate additional areas where either test is particularly useful.

References

1. Borer JS, Kent KM, Bacharach SL *et al.* Sensitivity, specificity and predictive accuracy of radionuclide cineangiography during exercise in patients with coronary artery disease. Circulation 1979;60:572–80.
2. Gibbons RJ, Lee KL, Cobb FR *et al.* Ejection fraction response to exercise in patients with chest pain, coronary artery disease and normal resting ventricular function. Circulation 1982;66:643–8.
3. Gibbons RJ. Equilibrium radionuclide angiography. In: Marcus ML, Schelbert HR, Skorton DJ, Wolf GL, editors. Cardiac imaging A companion to Braunwald's Heart Disease. Saunders: 1991, 1027–46.
4. Thrall JH, Froelich JW. Radionuclide ventriculography: Methods. In: Gerson MC. Cardiac Nuclear Medicine. New York: McGraw-Hill, 1987.
5. Manyari DE, Kostuk WJ. Left and right ventricular function at rest and during bicycle exercise in the supine and sitting positions in normal subjects and patients with coronary artery disease. Am J Cardiol 1983;51:36–42.

6. Currie PJ, Kelly MJ, Pitt A. Comparison of supine and erect bicycle exercise electrocardiography in coronary heart disease: accentuation of exercise-induced ischemic ST depression by supine position. Am J Cardiol 1983;52:1167–73.
7. Jones RH. Radionuclide angiocardiography. In: Marcus ML, Schelbert HR, Skorton DJ, Wolf GL, editors. Cardiac imaging A companion to Braunwald's Heart Disease. Saunders: 1991, 1006–26.
8. Austin EH, Cogg FR, Coleman RE, Jones RH. Prospective evaluation of radionuclide angiocardiography for the diagnosis of coronary artery disease. Am J Cardiol 1982;50:1212–6.
9. Gibbons RJ, Lee KL, Cobb F, Jones RH. Ejection fraction response to exercise in patients with chest pain and normal coronary arteriograms. Circulation 1981;64:952–7.
10. Gibbons RJ, Lee KL, Cobb FR *et al.* Ejection fraction response to exercise in patients with chest pain, coronary artery disease, and normal resting ventricular function. Circulation 1982;66:643–8.
11. Gibbons RJ, Lee KL, Pryer D *et al.* The use of radionuclide angiography in the diagnosis of coronary artery disease, a logistic regression analysis. Circulation 1983;68:740–6.
12. Jones RH, McEwan P, Newman GE *et al.* Accuracy of diagnosis of coronary artery disease by radionuclide measurement of left ventricular functionduring rest and exercise. Circulation 1981;64:586–601.
13. Rozanski A, Diamond GA, Forrester JS *et al.* Should the content of testing influence its interpretation? J Am Coll Cardiol 1986;7:17–24.
14. Rozanski A, Diamond GA, Forrester JS *et al.* The declining specificity of exercise radionuclide ventriculopathy. N Engl J Med 1983;309:518–22.
15. Port S, Cobb FR, Coleman RE, Jones RH. The effects of age on the response of the left ventricular ejection fraction to exercise. N Engl J Med 1980;303:1133–9.
16. Higgenbotham MB, Morris KG, Coleman RE, Cobb FR. Sex related differences in normal cardiac response to upright exercise. Circulation 1984;70:357–64.
17. Gerson MC. Myocardial perfusion imaging: Kinetics and planar methods. In: Gerson MC. Cardiac Nuclear Medicine. New York: McGraw-Hill, 1987.
18. Kiat H, Berman DS, Maddahi J *et al.* Late reversibility of tomographic myocardial Tl-201 defects: An accurate marker of myocardial viability. J Am Coll Cardiol 1988;12:1456–63.
19. Dilsizian V, Rocco TP, Freedman NM, Leon MB, Bonow RO. Enhanced detection of ischemic but viable myocardium by the reinjection of thallium after stress-redistribution imaging. N Engl J Med 1990;323:141–6.
20. Gould KL, Westcott RJ, Albro PC, Hamilton GW. Noninvasive assessment of coronary stenoses by myocardial imaging during pharmacologic coronary vasodilatation. II. Clinical methodology and feasibility. Am J Cardiol 1978;41:279–87.
21. Iskandrian AS, Heo J, Kong B, Lyons E. Effect of exercise level on the ability of thallium-201 tomographic imaging in detecting coronary artery disease: Analysis of 461 patients. J Am Coll Cardiol 1989;14:1477–86.
22. Kotler TS, Diamond GA. Exercise thallium-201 scintigraphy in the diagnosis and prognosis of coronary artery disease. Ann Intern Med 1990;113:684–702.
23. Fintel DJ, Links JM, Brinker JA, Frank TL, Parker M, Becker LC. Improved diagnostic performance of exercise thallium-201 single photon emission computed tomography over planar imaging in the diagnosis of coronary artery disease: A receiver operating characteristic analysis. J Am Coll Cardiol 1989;13:600–12.
24. Van Train KF, Maddahi J, Berman DS, Kiat H, Areeda J, Prigent F, Friedman J, and Participants of the Multicenter Trial. Quantitative analysis of tomographic stress thallium-201 myocardial scintigrams: A multicenter trial. J Nucl Med 1990;31:1168–79.
25. Lebowitz E, Greene MV, Fairchild R *et al.* Thallium-201 for medical use. J Nucl Med 1976;16:151–6.
26. Kahn JK, McGhie I, Akers MS *et al.* Quantitative rotational tomography with 201–Tl and 99 m-Tc 2–methoxy-isobutyl-isonitrile. A direct comparison in normal individuals and patients with coronary artery disease. Circulation 1989;79:1282–90.

27. Marwick T, Go RT, MacIntyre W *et al.* Comparison of myocardial perfusion imaging using positron emission tomography and single photon emission computed tomography: Frequency and causes of discrepant results. Eur Heart J 1991;12:1064–9.
28. Go R, Marwick T, MacIntyre W *et al.* A prospective comparison of rubidium-82. PET and thallium 201 SPECT myocardial perfusion imaging utilizing a single dipyridamole stress in the diagnosis of coronary artery disease. J Nucl Med 1990;331:1899–905.
29. Stewart R, Schwager M, Molina E *et al.* Comparison of rubidium-82 positron emission tomography and thallium-201 SPECT imaging for detection of coronary artery disease. Am J Cardiol 1991;67:1303–10.
30. Van Reet R, Quinones MA, Poliner LA *et al.* Comparison of two-dimensional echocardiography with gated radionuclide ventriculography in the evaluation of global and regional left ventricular function in acute myocardial infarction. J Am Coll Cardiol 1984;3:243–52.
31. Ginzton LE, Conant R, Brizendine M, Lee F, Mena I, Laks MM. Exercise subcostal two-dimensional echocardiography: A new method of segmental wall motion analysis. Am J Cardiol 1984;53:805–11.
32. Limacher MC, Quinones MA, Poliner LR, Nelson JG, Winters WL, Waggoner AD. Detection of coronary artery disease with exercise two-dimensional echocardiography: Description of a clinically applicable method and comparison with radionuclide ventriculography. Circulation 1983;67:1211–8.
33. Visser CA, van der Wieken RL, Kan G *et al.* Comparison of two-dimensional echocardiography with radionuclide angiography during dynamic exercise for the detection of coronary artery disease. Am Heart J 1983;106:528–34.
34. Crawford MH, Petru MA, Amon KW, Sorensen SG, Vance WS. Comparitive value of 2–dimensional echocardiography and radionuclide angiography for quantitating changes in left ventricular performance during exercise limited by angina pectoris. Am J Cardiol 1984;53:42–6.
35. Dehmer GJ, Firth BG, Hillis LD *et al.* Alterations in left ventricle volume and ejection fraction at rest and during exercise in patients with aortic regurgitation. Am J Cardiol 1981;48:17–27.
36. Marwick T, Torelli J, Underwood D, MacIntyre WJ. Metabolic evidence of ischemia following high- and low-dose dipyridamole stress [abstract]. J Nucl Med 1992;33:866.
37. Lattanzi F, Picano E, Bolognese L *et al.* Inhibition of dipyridamole-induced ischemia by antianginal therapy in humans. Circulation 1991;83:1256–62.
38. Leppo J, Boucher CA, Okada RD, Newell JB, Strauss HW, Pohost GM. Serial thallium-201 myocardial imaging after dipyridamole infusion: Diagnostic utility in detection of coronary stenoses and relation to regional wall motion. Circulation 1982;66:649–57.
39. Maurer G, Nanda NC. Two dimensional echocardiographic evaluation of exercise-induced left and right ventricular asynergy: Correlation with thallium scanning. Am J Cardiol 1981;48:720–7.
40. Galanti G, Sciagra R, Comeglio M *et al.* Diagnostic accuracy of peak exercise echocardiography in coronary artery disease: Comparison with thallium-201 myocardial scintigraphy. Am Heart J 1991;122:1609–16.
41. Pozzoli MM, Fioretti PM, Salustri A, Reijs AE, Roelandt JR. Exercise echocardiography and technetium-99 m MIBI single photon emission computed tomography in the detection of coronary artery disease. Am J Cardiol 1991;67:350–5.
42. Salustri A, Pozzoli MM, Hermans W *et al.* Relationship between exercise echocardiography and perfusion single photon emission computed tomography in patients with single vessel coronary artery disease. Am Heart J 1992;124:75–83.
43. Quinones MA, Verani MS, Haichin RM, Mahmarian JJ, Suarez J, Zoghbi WA. Exercise echocardiography versus Tl-201 single photon emission computed tomography in evaluation of coronary artery disease. Analysis of 292 patients. Circulation 1992;85:1026–31.
44. Marwick T, D'Hondt AM, Baudhuin T *et al.* Optimal use of Dobutamine Stress for the Detection and Evaluation of Coronary Artery Disease: Combination with Echocardiography, Scintigraphy or Both? J Am Coll Cardiol 1993;22:159–67.

45. Labowitz AJ, Pearson AC, Chaitman BR. Doppler and two-dimensional echocardiographic assessment of left ventricular function before and after intravenous dipyridamole stress testing for detection of coronary artery disease. Am J Cardiol 1988;62:1180–5.
46. Grayburn PA, Popma JJ, Pryor SL, Walker BS, Simon TR, Smitherman TC. Comparison of dipyridamole Doppler echocardiography to thallium-201 imaging and quantitative coronary arteriography in the assessment of coronary artery disease. Am J Cardiol 1989;63:1315–20.
47. Perin EC, Moore W, Blume M, Hernandez G, Dhekne R, DeCastro M. Comparison of dipyridamole echocardiography with dipyridamole thallium scintigraphy for the diagnosis of myocardial ischemia. Clin Nucl Med 1991;16:417–20.
48. Simonetti I, Rezai K, Rossen JD *et al.* Physiological assessment of sensitivity of noninvasive testing for coronary artery disease. Circulation 1991;83(Suppl III):43–9.
49. Parodi O, Bisi G, Cassucci R *et al.* Clinical efficacy of Tc-99 m MIBI scintigraphy associated to echocardiography and dipyridamole test for the detection of coronary artery disease: A multicenter study [abstract]. Circulation 1989;80:II–620.
50. Marwick T, Willemart B, D'Hondt AM *et al.* Selection of the optimal non-exercise stress for the evaluation of ischemic regional myocardial dysfunction and malperfusion: Comparison of dobutamine and adenosine using echocardiography and Tc-99 m MIBI single photon emission computed tomography. Circulation 1993;87:345–54.
51. Marwick T, Salcedo E, Covalesky R, Stewart WJ. Comparison of stress echocardiography and thallium tomography – Analysis of discrepant results [abstract]. J Am Soc Echo 1990;3:226.
52. Marwick T, Stewart WJ, Salcedo EE. Diagnosis of coronary artery disease using exercise echocardiography and positron emission tomography: Comparison and analysis of discrepant results. J Am Soc Echo 1992;5:231–8.
53. Liu P, Keiss MC, Okada RD *et al.* The persistent defect on exercise thallium imaging and its fate after myocardial revascularization: does it represent scar or ischemia? Am Heart J 1985;110:996–1001.
54. Kerber RE, Marcus ML, Ehrhardt J, Wilson R, Abbout FM. Correlation between echocardiographically demonstrated dyskinesis and regional myocardial perfusion. Circulation 1975;52:1097–104.
55. De Puey EG, Garcia EV. Optimal specificity of thallium-201 SPECT through recognition of imaging artifacts. J Nucl Med 1989;30:441–9.
56. DePuey EG, Guertler-Krawczynska E, Robbins WL. Thallium-201 SPECT in coronary disease patients with left bundle branch block. J Nucl Med 1988;29:1479–85.
57. Burns RJ, Galligan L, Wright LM, Lawand S, Burke RK, Gladstone PJ. Improved specificity of myocardial thallium-201 single-photon emission computed tomography in patients with left bundle branch block by dipyridamole. Am J Cardiol 1991;68:504–8.
58. Matzer L, Kiat H, Friedman JR, van Train K, Maddahi J, Berman DS. A new approach to the assessment of tomographic thallium-201 scintigraphy in patients with left bundle branch block. J Am Coll Cardiol 1991;17:1309–17.
59. Bramlet DA, Morris KG, Coleman RE, Albert D, Cobb FR. Effects of rate-dependent left bundle branch block on global and regional left ventricular function. Circulation 1983;67:1059–65.
60. Rowe DW, DePuey EG, Sonnemaker RE, Hall RJ, Burdine JA. Left ventricular performance during exercise in patients with left bundle branch block: Evaluation by gated radionuclide ventriculography. Am Heart J 1983;105:66–71.
61. DePuey EG, Guertler-Krawczynska E, Perkins JV, Robbins WL, Whelchel JD, Clements SD. Alterations in myocardial thallium-201 distribution in patients with chronic systemic hypertension undergoing single-photon emission computed tomography. Am J Cardiol 1988;62:234–8.
62. Houghton TL, Frank MJ, Carr AA, VonDohlen TW, Prisant LM. Relations among impaired coronary flow reserve, left ventricular hypertrophy, and thallium perfusion defects in hypertensive patients without obstructive coronary artery disease. J Am Coll Cardiol 1990;15:43–51.

63. Mueller T, Marcus M, Kerber R, Young Y, Barnes R, Abboud F. Effect of renal hypertension and left ventricular hypertrophy on the coronary circulation in dogs. Circ Res 1978;42:543–9.
64. O'Keefe DD, Hoffman JIE, Cheitlin R, O'Neill MJ, Allard JR, Shapkin E. Coronary blood flow in experimental canine left ventricular hypertrophy. Circ Res 1978;43:43–51.
65. Malik AB, Abe T, O'Kane H, Geha AS. Cardiac function, coronary flow, and oxygen consumption in stable left ventricular hypertrophy. Am J Physiol 1973;225:186–91.
66. Bache RJ, Vrobel TR, Arentzen CE, Ring WS. Effect of maximum coronary vasodilation on transmural myocardial perfusion during tachycardia in dogs with left ventricular hypertrophy. Circ Res 1981;49:742–50.
67. Rembert J, Kleinman L, Fedor J, Wechsler A, Greenfield J. Myocardial blood flow distribution in concentric left ventricular hypertrophy. J Clin Invest 1978;62:379–86.
68. O'Keefe DD, Hoffman JIE, Cheitlin R, O'Neill MJ, Allard JR, Shapkin E. Coronary blood flow in experimental canine left ventricular hypertrophy. Circ Res 1978;43:43–51.
69. Goldstein RA, Haynie M. Limited myocardial perfusion reserve in patients with left ventricular hypertrophy. J Nucl Med 1990;31:225–8.
70. Marwick T, Cook SA, Lafont A, Underwood DA, Salcedo EE. Influence of left ventricular mass on the diagnostic accuracy of myocardial perfusion imaging using positron emission tomography with dipyridamole stress. J Nucl Med 1991;32:2221–6.

8. Use of Stress Echocardiography for Assessment of Interventions and Medical Treatments

The previous sections have dealt with issues relating to the performance of stress echocardiography for the diagnosis of coronary artery disease. However, the chronic nature of this illness mandates the careful follow-up of patients, to identify the progression of disease or the development of complications. Functional tests are well suited to monitoring the progress of patients in these respects. This chapter will review data pertaining to the efficacy of stress echocardiography for the follow-up of patients after coronary bypass surgery, coronary angioplasty, and medical therapy of ischemic heart disease.

8.1 Use of Stress Echocardiography after Coronary Artery Bypass Surgery

Despite the efficacy of surgical revascularization of the myocardium for the relief of angina, the process of bypassing coronary stenoses with vein grafts is essentially a temporary, palliative measure. The recurrence of angina after coronary artery bypass surgery is frequent, occurring in 38% of patients in the 6 year interval after surgery [1]. This recurrence reflects both the progression of native vessel disease and graft failure. Indeed, one year after operation, the bypass occlusion rate varies from 10 to 31%, and significant stenoses are present in 10% of vein grafts at 18 months [2–5]. The evaluation of these patients for recurrent ischemia therefore constitutes an important clinical challenge, particularly in the light of the high prevalence of coronary bypass surgery.

Unfortunately, ischemia may not be reliably detected using conventional criteria in this group of patients. Chest pain is both frequent and difficult to interpret. The high prevalence of musculoskeletal pains causes chest discomfort to be non-specific for the presence of coronary stenoses [6]. Routine exercise testing has suboptimal sensitivity in this population, as many patients in this group show features such as repolarization abnormalities which compromise its interpretation [6–8]. The sensitivity of thallium imaging for the detection of progressive coronary disease has also been limited [8–12]. Some of the problems of conventional scintigraphic imaging (photon attenuation, contrast resolution, and the distinction of ischemia from scar) may be circumvented using positron emission tomography. However, while this

T.H. Marwick, Stress Echocardiography, 139–145.

technique reliably identifies recurrent atherosclerosis after bypass surgery [13], it is not a clinically feasible test on the grounds of cost and availability.

Stress echocardiography may be an attractive alternative to the current approaches for the diagnosis of recurrent ischemia in post-bypass surgery patients. As discussed in Chapter 5, the sensitivity of stress echocardiography exceeds that of the stress ECG. Moreover, stress echocardiography may avoid the problem of delayed thallium redistribution, which, because of the high prevalence of myocardial infarction among patients undergoing bypass surgery, is a frequent source of ambiguity between ischemia and scar in this population. Recent studies support the accuracy of exercise echocardiography in post-bypass patients. Sawada [14] studied 42 patients at a mean interval of 6 years after surgery, reporting a feasibility of 90%, a sensitivity of 94% and a specificity of 83%. In a group of 125 patients [15], the feasibility of stress echocardiography was 100%, with a sensitivity of 98% and specificity of 92%, both being superior to the results of ST segment analysis. Williams [16] found stress echocardiography to have a sensitivity of 95% and specificity of 87% in 34 patients. Unlike the situation of native coronary disease, the use of a multivariate exercise score (see Chapter 5) did not appear to enhance the results of ST segment analysis. All studies indicate that the technique reliably identifies the site and extent of recurrent or persisting coronary disease.

Similarly, the results of high-dose dipyridamole echocardiography normalize early after bypass surgery [17]. However, data pertaining to the efficacy of pharmacologic stress echocardiography for the late detection of recurrent coronary disease are more scant.

8.2 Stress Echocardiographic Evaluation of Patients Undergoing Coronary Angioplasty

Since its inception over a decade ago, percutaneous transluminal coronary angioplasty (PTCA) has proven to be a safe and effective means of treating coronary stenoses [18]. As stress echocardiography is a readily repeatable non-invasive investigation, it may have a role in the selection, early evaluation and late follow-up of patients undergoing this procedure.

The accepted indications for PTCA vary on a idiosyncratic basis, but an obvious precondition is the presence of myocardial ischemia. This is generally not in question when PTCA is performed for the treatment of unstable angina, but may be a consideration in the management of chronic angina. In the current environment of cost-control, the demonstration of ischemia within the territory of a potentially angioplastiable vessel may be used to justify such an intervention. Not surprisingly, stress echocardiography has been almost uniformly positive in series of patients selected by other means to undergo PTCA [19–21].

While PTCA is known to relieve angina promptly in most patients, the seeds of recurrent angina – incomplete revascularization and restenosis – are to some extent present following the initial procedure. Although restenosis is a heterogeneous syndrome, some such complications actually reflect residual stenosis, which may be difficult to recognize on post-PTCA angiograms because of apparent improvement of luminal dimensions secondary to extravasation of contrast into the media due to plaque fissuring and dissection. Indeed, quantitative angiographic methods [22] have shown that the absolute diameter of the vessel following the procedure is independently predictive of this problem. Studies examining the prognostic significance of stress echocardiographic findings early after PTCA [20,21] have shown that a persistently positive test reliably predicts the recurrence of angina. Moreover, this functional evaluation appears to avoid the problem of delayed normalization of coronary flow reserve in the immediate post-PTCA period, defined by invasive means [23], and evident at thallium imaging [24]. Direct comparison of dobutamine stress perfusion scintigraphy and echocardiography in 26 patients within 24 hours of PTCA showed residual stress perfusion defects in 5 patients (19%), only one of whom had abnormal function by stress echocardiography [25]. In summary, there may be some benefit in functional evaluation of patients after PTCA, and these preliminary data suggest that, for this purpose, echocardiography is the test of choice.

At subsequent follow-up, restenosis remains the single greatest problem besetting PTCA, occurring in approximately one third of patients and segments [22]. In practical terms, the need for a test to identify recurrent disease late after the procedure far exceeds the role of investigations for selection and early evaluation of PTCA. Stress echocardiography has proven to effectively identify patients with restenosis [21,26,27]. At late post-PTCA follow-up, results have been shown to correlate well with those of perfusion scintigraphy [28,29].

8.3 Stress Echocardiography and the Effects of Drug Therapy

As stress-induced wall motion abnormalities are based upon the development of myocardial ischemia, it might be anticipated that the results of stress echocardiography may be modulated by the treatment of ischemia. While this has implications for the diagnostic use of stress echocardiography, it may also offer a role for this test in the evaluation of drug therapy. In this respect, stress echocardiography can offer more comprehensive data than merely detecting the presence or absence of myocardial ischemia. The extent of ischemia may be assessed from the severity of global left ventricular dysfunction, as well as the number of segments involved. The severity of ischemia may estimated by use of a wall motion score, or by the amount of stress required to induce an ischemic response – most readily measured as the duration of stress.

The effects of anti-anginal therapy upon the results of stress echocardiography have been studied most effectively using dipyridamole stress. In a placebo-controlled cross-over study [30] of 57 patients with significant coronary disease (defined by >70% diameter stenoses), 91% developed echocardiographic evidence of ischemia off therapy, but only 65% became ischemic on therapy ($p < 0.01$). This effect was most marked for the combination of beta-blockers and nifedipine (33% sensitivity vs 100% in the control group), and was roughly equally represented in patients on beta-blockers (sensitivity 67%), calcium antagonists (sensitivity 62%) and a calcium antagonist-nitrate combination (71%). These effects paralleled the influence of drug therapy on the results of exercise testing – the number of positive tests being 47% on therapy and 70% off therapy. In those patients whose stress echocardiograms remained positive for ischemia, the time until the onset of ischemia significantly lengthened with therapy, again matched by a similar enhancement of exercise time. Finally, therapy was associated with a reduction of the wall motion score index, though this alteration did not correlate well with alteration of exercise time, possibly because of the use of ischemia as a test endpoint (thereby blunting the possible maximal wall motion score). Recently, these findings have been reproduced using beta blocker therapy alone [31].

The above findings support the role of stress echocardiography for the evaluation of drug therapy. However, the use of dipyridamole for this purpose does not reflect the usual mechanism of ischemia due to increased oxygen demand. Indeed, as the main effects of dipyridamole pertain to coronary steal, it is presumably the collateral-related effects of calcium antagonists and nitrates which are tested with this protocol. Similarly, the protection of subendocardial flow by beta-blockade presumably constitutes the mechanism of the control of dipyridamole-induced ischemia with this drug.

Thus, an approach which evaluated the effects of drug therapy on exercise- or dobutamine-induced ischemia may be more attractive from the standpoint of evaluation of anti-anginal therapy. Unfortunately, such data are sparse. Iliceto [32] has reported improvement of the wall motion score index during atrial pacing, with gallopamil therapy. The effects of beta-adrenoceptor blockade on dobutamine stress echocardiography are disputed. No effect of beta blockade on the accuracy of dobutamine echocardiography was reported by Salustri [33], but a reduction of myocardial ischemia due to treatment may have been concealed by a higher prevalence of coronary disease in patients on beta-blocker therapy. We found that beta-blocker therapy on the day of the test, combined with the performance of submaximal tests, correlated with false negative findings [34]. However, it is uncertain whether a reduction of dobutamine echocardiography sensitivity in this situation would reflect the anti-ischemic action of beta-blockade, rather than an inhibitory effect upon receptor stimulation.

At exercise echocardiography, a submaximal heart-rate response has been shown to correlate with false negative results [35], and beta-blockade is certainly a potent source of submaximal heart-rate responses. However, no direct effect of drug therapy on exercise echocardiography results has been reported, and indeed no placebo controlled study of the effects of medical therapy on exercise-induced wall motion abnormalities has been published to date.

8.4 Evaluation of Heart Transplants Using Stress Echocardiography

Following heart transplantation, patients are prone to accelerated atherogenesis in the graft coronary vasculature. Moreover, as ischemia in the denervated heart may be clinically silent, intensive follow-up – including routine follow-up angiography – is often performed to identify it. The routine stress ECG has not found wide following for this purpose because the resting ECG is often uninterpretable for ischemia, and because coronary disease is often mild. These considerations might suggest a role for stress echocardiography in post-transplant surveillance.

The usefulness of dipyridamole echocardiography for this purpose has recently been reported by Ciliberto [36]. The test proved to have 100% specificity for those with normal coronaries, and had a sensitivity of 87% for detection of >50% stenoses, the latter being the only patients with cardiac events at early (9 month) follow-up. We compared the feasibility and specificity of exercise ECG, echocardiography and perfusion imaging in 35 patients without coronary disease at an interval of 33 ± 16 months after transplantation. The exercise ECG was uninterpretable due to resting ST segment abnormalities in 14 patients (feasibility 60%), and 19 of the remaining 21 had a normal test (specificity 90%). Exercise echocardiography could not be performed in 1 patient (feasibility 97%), though 7 others had studies of poor quality due to abnormal cardiac orientation. Abnormal septal motion was present in 20 patients at rest, but no stress-induced wall motion abnormalities were observed (specificity 100%). All patients had interpretable MIBI-SPECT images (feasibility 100%); resting perfusion defects were present in 3 patients, and 3 had a stress-induced defect (specificity 91%). Thus, in the search for coronary graft disease, the exercise ECG is often not feasible, and exercise echocardiography (which may be technically difficult) or MIBI are highly specific for coronary disease [37].

References

1. Gershlick AH, Lyons JP, Wright JEC, Sturridge MF, Layton CA, Balcon R. Long-term clinical outcome of coronary surgery and assessment of the benefit obtained with postoperative aspirin and dipyridamole. Br Heart J 1988;60:111–6.
2. Murphy ML, Hulgren HN, Detre K *et al*. Treatment of chronic stable angina: a preliminary report of survival data in the randomized Veterans Administration cooperative Study. N Engl J Med 1977;297:621–7.

3. European Coronary Surgery Study Group. Coronary artery bypass surgery in stable angina pectoris: survival at two years. Lancet 1979;i:589–93.
4. Principal Investigators of CASS and their Associates. National Heart, Lung and Blood Institute Coronary Artery Surgery Study. Circulation 1981;63 (suppl I)I.1–I.81.
5. Hamby RI, Aintablain A, Handler M *et al.* Aortocoronary saphenous vein bypass grafts: Long-term patency, morphology and blood flow in patients with patent grafts early after surgery. Circulation 1979;60:901–9.
6. Robinson PS, Williams BT, Webb-Peploe MM, Crowther A, Coltart DJ. Thallium-201 myocardial imaging in assessment of results of aortocoronary bypass surgery. Br Heart J 1979;42:455–62.
7. Greenberg BH, Hart R, Botvinick EH *et al.* Thallium-201 myocardial perfusion scintigraphy to evaluate patients after coronary bypass surgery. Am J Cardiol 1978;42:167–76.
8. Hirzel HO, Nuesch K, Sialer G, Horst W, Krayenbuehl HP. Thallium-201 exercise myocardial imaging to evaluate myocardial perfusion after coronary artery bypass surgery. Br Heart J 1980;43:426–35.
9. Wainwright RJ, Brennand-Roper DA, Maisey MN, Sowton E. Exercise thallium-201 myocardial scintigraphy in the follow-up of aortocoronary bypass graft surgery. Br Heart J 1980;43:56–66.
10. Pfisterer M, Emmenegger H, Schmitt HE *et al.* Accuracy of serial myocardial perfusion scintigraphy with thallium-201 for prediction of graft patency early and late after coronary artery bypass surgery. Circulation 1982;66:1017–24.
11. Iskandrian AS, Haaz W, Segal BL, Kane SA. Exercise thallium-201 scintigraphy in evaluating aortocoronary bypass surgery. Chest 1981;80:11–5.
12. Paolillo V, Iazzolino E, Varetto T *et al.* Myocardial scintigraphy with thallium-201 in the evaluation of aortocoronary bypass patients. G Ital Cardiol 1987;17:947–56.
13. Marwick T, Lafont A, Go RT *et al.* Diagnostic accuracy of positron emission tomography in the identification of recurrent ischemia after coronary artery bypass surgery. Int J Cardiol 1992;35:33–41.
14. Sawada SG, Judson WE, Ryan T, Armstrong WF, Feigenbaum H. Upright bicycle exercise echocardiography after coronary artery bypass grafting. Am J Cardiol 1989;64:1123–9.
15. Crouse LJ, Vacek JL, Beauchamp GD, Porter CB, Rosamond TL, Kramer PH. Exercise echocardiography after coronary artery bypass grafting. Am J Cardiol 1992;70:572–6.
16. Williams J, O'Gorman D, Foale RA, Marwick T. Stress echocardiography is superior to ST segment and multivariate ECG analysis for detection of ischemia after coronary artery bypass grafting [Abstract]. Eur Heart J 1993 (in press).
17. Biagini A, Maffei S, Baroni M *et al.* Early assessment of coronary reserve after bypass surgery by dipyridamole transesophageal echocardiographic stress test. Am Heart J 1990;120:1097–101.
18. Holmes DR, Holubkov R, Vlietstra Re *et al.* for the NHLBI PTCA Registry. Comparison of complications during percutaneous transluminal coronary angioplasty from 1977 to 1981 and 1985 to 1986; The NHLBI PTCA Registry. J Am Coll Cardiol 1988;12:1149–55.
19. Broderick T, Sawada S, Armstrong WF *et al.* Improvement in rest and exercise-induced wall motion abnormalities after coronary angioplasty: An exercise echocardiographic study. J Am Coll Cardiol 1990;15:591–9.
20. Massa D, Pirelli S, Gara E *et al.* Exercise testing and dipyridamole echocardiography test before and 48h after successful coronary angioplasty: Prognostic implications. Eur Heart J 1989;10(Suppl G):13–7.
21. Picano E, Pirelli S, Marzilli M *et al.* Usefulness of high-dose dipyridamole echocardiography test in coronary angioplasty. Circulation 1989;80:807–15.
22. Renkin J, Melin JA, Robert A *et al.* Detection of restenosis after successful coronary angioplasty: Improved clinical decision making with use of a logistic regression model combining procedural and follow-up variables. J Am Coll Cardiol 1990;16:1333–40.
23. Laarman GJ, Serruys PW, Suryapranata H *et al.* Inability of coronary blood flow reserve

measurements to assess the efficacy of coronary angioplasty in the first 24 hours in unselected patients. Am Heart J 1991 122:631–9

24. Manyari DE, Knudtson M, Kloiber R, Roth D Sequential thallium-201 myocardial perfusion studies after successful PTCA. Delayed resolution of exercise-induced scintigraphic abnormalities. Circulation 1988;77.86–95
25 Marwick T Baudhuin T Willemart W D'Hondt AM, Wijns W Melin J Differential alteration of regional left ventricular function and perfusion responses to cardiac stress early after coronary angioplasty [abstract] Eur Heart J 1992,13(Suppl):404.
26. Pirelli S, Danzi GB Alberti A *et al.* Comparison of usefulness of high-dose dipyridamole echocardiography and exercise electrocardiography for detection of asymptomatic restenosis after coronary angioplasty Am J Cardiol 1991;67 1335–8.
27 Aboul-Enein H, Bengtson JR, Adams DB *et al* Effect of the degree of effort on exercise echocardiography for the detection of restenosis after coronary artery angioplasty Am Heart J 1991 122:430–7
28. Fioretti PM, Pozzoli MMA, Ilmer B *et al.* Exercise echocardiography versus thallium-201 SPECT for assessing patients before and after PTCA. Eur Heart J 1992,13:213–9
29 McNeill AJ Fioretti PM, El-Said EM, Salustri A, de Feyter PJ Roelandt JR. Dobutamine stress echocardiography before and after coronary angioplasty Am J Cardiol 1992;69·740–5
30. Lattanzi F Picano E, Bolognese L *et al* Inhibition of dipyridamole-induced ischemia by antianginal therapy in humans. Correlation with exercise echocardiography Circulation 1991,83·1256–62.
31 Ferrara N Longobardi G Nicolino A *et al.* Effect of beta-adrenoceptor blockade on dipyridamole-induced myocardial asynergies in coronary artery disease. Am J Cardiol 1992;70:724–7
32. Iliceto S Caiati C, Tota F Rizzon P The importance of stress-induced cardiac wall motion abnormalities in the evaluation of drug intervention. Drugs 1992;43(Suppl 1 :33–6.
33 Salustri A, Fioretti PR, Pozzoli MMA, McNeill AJ Roelandt JR. Dobutamine stress echocardiography· its role in the diagnosis of coronary artery disease. Eur Heart J 1992,13:70–7
34. Marwick T D'Hondt AM, Baudhuin T *et al* Optimal use of dobutamine stress for the detection and evaluation of coronary artery disease. Combination with echocardiography scintigraphy or both? J Am Coll Cardiol 1993;22.159–67
35 Marwick T Nemec J Pashkow F Stewart WJ Salcedo E. Accuracy and limitations of exercise echocardiography in a routine clinical setting. J Am Coll Cardiol 1992,19·74–81
36. Ciliberto GR, Massa D Mangiavacchi M *et al.* High-dose dipyridamole echocardiography test in coronary artery disease after heart transplantation. Eur Heart J 1993;14:48–52.
37 Marwick T D'Hondt AM, Baudhuin T *et al.* Choice of exercise ECG perfusion scintigraphy or exercise echocardiography for detection of graft vessel atherosclerosis [abstract] Br Heart J 1993 (in press

9. Prognostic Value of Stress Echocardiography

Previous chapters have concentrated upon the ability of stress echocardiography to predict the presence of significant coronary artery disease. This approach permits the comparison of this test and various other non-invasive methodologies, using angiographic stenosis as the reference standard. However, this standard may be difficult to accurately define [1], and may not correlate with functional indices of coronary flow [2]. Consequently, the clinical value of identifying moderate (but "significant") coronary stenoses may reasonably be questioned.

An alternative approach is to use indices of patient outcome to judge the efficacy of testing. This has the merit of being more directly pertinent to patient care; our attempts to identify coronary disease are made so as to predict and/or treat the sequelae of the disease – myocardial ischemia, infarction and death. Thus, a test providing reliable prognostic information is not only useful to the patient (for making plans for the future), but by identifying high risk patients, may help select individuals for intervention. This chapter will examine the usefulness of stress echocardiography for the prediction of major cardiac events in patients with chronic stable angina, for prognostication in patients after myocardial infarction, and for forecasting cardiac complications at major non-cardiac (vascular) surgery.

9.1 Assessment of Prognosis in Patients with Stable Coronary Disease

The average annual mortality among all patients with chronic stable angina was low – only 4% – even in the days before widespread use of modern therapeutic regimens [3]. Some clinical data (pertaining to the severity of angina, a history of hypertension or prior infarction, and resting ST segment depression) may identify subgroups at higher and lower risk [4]. However, in patients without prior infarction, coronary angiography has provided more powerful prognostic data – the detection of three-vessel or left main coronary disease identifies subgroups with 5 year mortalities of 15% or 43%, respectively [4,5]. The coronary anatomy carries prognostic significance because it determines the extent of myocardial ischemia. Hence, the only modest ability of stress echocardiography (or any non-invasive test), for the prediction of the exact coronary anatomy [6,7] may not compromise the prognostic rel-

T.H. Marwick, Stress Echocardiography, 147–162.

evance of its results, provided that the extent of ischemia is identified. On these grounds, exercise capacity and ST segment depression at exercise testing both offer important prognostic information in patients with stable coronary disease [8], as do the results of nuclear ventriculography and thallium imaging [9,10].

Useful prognostic data might therefore be expected of stress echocardiography, which identifies the presence, extent and severity of myocardial ischemia. Unfortunately, with the development of the technique at the same time as the development of readily available coronary revascularization at coronary angioplasty, natural history data are sparse with respect to positive test results, as many such patients proceed to intervention. The exception is the study of Corday [11], who followed 16 patients with an abnormal stress ECG and wall motion abnormalities for a mean period of 19 months, over which time, 6 (38%) suffered cardiac events.

The prognostic value of a negative stress echocardiogram is equally important, as it addresses an important limitation of comparisons with coronary angiography – the issue of post-test selection bias [12]. This arises if all patients in a series do not submit to angiography. The non-invasive test then appears to be sensitive (as those with positive tests are most likely to undergo angiography), but questions remain as to the outcome of those with negative results who tend not to be investigated further. The consequences of "false negative" studies are best addressed by follow-up of patients at some time interval after the test. Studies performed over several years of follow-up have shown patients with normal exercise electrocardiography results to have a benign prognosis [8]. Similar findings have been reported for patients having normal thallium-201 perfusion scintigraphy [13] or normal radionuclide ventriculography [10]. Few data are available to document the prognosis of individuals with a normal exercise echocardiogram. Corday [11] recorded no cardiac events over a 19 month period in patients with a normal exercise echocardiogram. Sawada [14] followed 148 such patients over a period of 28 ± 9 months, and found only 6 to have had cardiac events, all of which occurred in those patients who exercised submaximally (<85% age-predicted maximum heart-rate or <6 METS). These "events" comprised 4 patients requiring coronary revascularization, and 2 patients suffering myocardial infarction, giving a likelihood of myocardial infarction in patients with a negative exercise echocardiogram of 0.85% per year. However, the study population was one characterized by a low probability of coronary disease (39%), a high prevalence of females (almost 50%), and a mean age of 53 years. Other institutions, especially in Europe, might expect to see an older group of patients, fewer females, and a higher probability of coronary artery disease. No data are available regarding the prognostic value of the stress echocardiogram in such a population.

In those patients who are unable to exercise, preliminary data on pharmacologic stress echocardiography have also shown negative tests to herald an excellent prognosis. Picano [15] compared the prognostic implications of clinical features, the resting ECG and dipyridamole stress echocardiography in 539 patients. Cardiac events occurred in 83 of 204 patients (41%) with wall motion abnormalities occurring at low dose, 21 of 82 patients (26%) with high dose positivity, and 14 of 253 patients (6%) with normal echocardiography results. In a univariate analysis, a positive dipyridamole echocardiogram was the strongest predictor of death and hard events, followed by ECG changes and stress-induced angina. Positive dipyridamole echocardiography and angina were also the stongest predictors of hard events in a multivariate model. Furthermore, a sub-analysis of 341 patients with exercise ECG and coronary angiography findings demonstrated a positive stress echocardiogram to remain the best predictor of cardiac events.

Few data are available to address the prognostic value of dobutamine echocardiography. In a study of 291 patients [16], 1.3% of 76 patients with a normal dobutamine echocardiogram suffered a myocardial infarction over a mean follow-up of 15 months, with no cardiac deaths occurring in this group. Two of 39 patients with inducible ischemia (5%) suffered myocardial infarction and cardiac death. Those with ischemia and previous infarction had respective incidences of 9% and 19%.

9.2 Use of Stress Echocardiography to Assess Prognosis after Myocardial Infarction

The frequency of cardiac events in the first year after myocardial infarction has been reported to vary from 5 to 10% – higher than that associated with chronic stable angina [17]. The major determinants of adverse sequellae are the amount of infarcted myocardium (actual damage) and the extent of jeopardized myocardium (possible damage). The prognostic influence of myocardial dysfunction after myocardial infarction may be determined from the ejection fraction [18], from an analogous wall motion score index [19], or from the extent of the resting thallium defect [20]. The influence of ischemia is usually apparent from the stress ECG [21], perfusion [22] or wall motion imaging [23] during exercise or other stressors. Using a stepwise approach, about 20% of patients may be identified as being at very high risk (due to irreversible left ventricular dysfunction), 30% to be at moderate risk (on the basis of ongoing ischemia), and 50% at low risk [24].

No consensus exists regarding the optimal investigation of post-infarction patients. Preliminary risk stratification is possible using clinical data [25]. It is thus possible to identify groups at particularly low risk, in whom further investigations are not justified upon Bayesian grounds – indeed, the situation is analogous to that of diagnostic investigation in patients with a low pretest probability of coronary disease. Nonetheless, exercise testing is almost uniformly performed – partly because the presence of ongoing ischemia offers the prospect of intervention, and partly because exercise testing offers an important source of reassurance, which is important in rehabilitation. A negative exercise ECG [21] indicates a favorable prognosis, with a 2% mortality in the year after infarction, compared with a 27% mortality with a positive test. However, while the routine exercise ECG is a reasonable first test for prognostic stratification in post-infarct patients, it has important shortcomings. These include its inability to identify the site and extent of coronary disease, and its dependence on the patient's exercise capacity – such that patients with left ventricular dysfunction may fail to develop ischemia because their exercise capacity is too low. The need to overcome these issues, as well as to quantify the extent of left ventricular dysfunction, have driven the use of functional imaging after myocardial infarction. The prognostic data obtainable from thallium imaging [pertaining to not only the presence and extent of ischemia, but also the extent and severity of the total perfusion defect and evidence of stress-induced left ventricular failure) has been shown to more effectively identify high cardiac risk than exercise parameters or even coronary angiography [22]. Debate continues regarding the optimal combination of non-invasive studies. A recent comparison of the ability of exercise ECG, resting echocardiography, nuclear ventriculography and thallium imaging to predict both severe and total post-infarction complications, has suggested that the optimal approach is a combination of thallium imaging and nuclear ventriculography [26]. However, this study did not include stress echocardiography.

The echocardiographic identification of jeopardized myocardium may be divided into the detection of peri-infarct ischemia ("homozonal dyssynergy"), multivessel disease ("heterozonal dyssynergy") and residual viable myocardium in the infarct zone (Figure 9.1) – features which may be demonstrated at dobutamine or dipyridamole echocardiography. Moreover, stress echocardiography offers the ability to determine both the extent of left ventricular damage (on the resting images) and the extent of jeopardized myocardium (on stress images), using a single test. As the echocardiographic calculation of ejection fraction is based upon the assumption of a geometric ventricular shape, which is inappropriate after myocardial infarction, evaluation of left ventricular function is better made using a wall motion score [19].

Studies addressing the prognostic value of stress echocardiography after myocardial infarction are summarized in Table 9.1 [27–32]. The sensitivity for the recognition of ischemia at a distance was around 80%, and its specificity was around 90% [27,29], being comparable with the ability of scintigraphy to recognize multivessel disease in patients late after infarction (discussed in Chapter 3). In the series examining exercise stress, the sensitivity of a new wall motion abnormality (63 to 80%) and its specificity (65 to 76%) exceeded the sensitivity and specificity of ST segment depression for the prediction of cardiac events. In contrast to these results, rest and stress ejection fractions predicted multivessel disease [27] and cardiac events [28,29] less effectively than regional wall motion abnormalities. Moreover, the prognostic power of the stress echocardiography data was found to exceed that

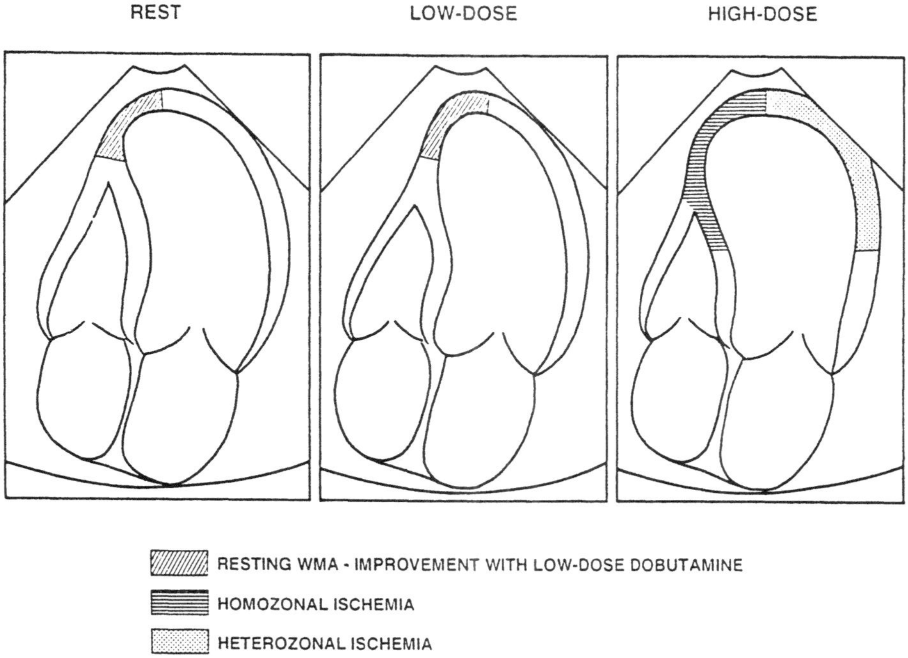

Figure 9.1. Schematic diagrams of apical 4–chamber views of the heart following a left anterior descending territory infarction, demonstrating a wall motion abnormality (WMA) at rest, with improvement of function during low-dose dobutamine therapy (denoting viability). At high doses of dobutamine, homozonal ischemia develops in this and adjacent tissue, as well as heterozonal ischemia in the left circumflex territory.

of clinical and exercise parameters, when compared in univariate and multivariate analyses [28].

While exercise testing is useful in reassuring patients about their ability to resume usual activities after myocardial infarction, and although exercise parameters are well known to carry independent prognostic information, there are nonetheless obvious attractions to the use of non-exercise techniques in the post-infarction population. Many recurrent ischemic events occur early after infarction, and a technique which can be brought to the bedside offers the possibility of identifying and treating "at risk" patients before events occur. Dipyridamole, dobutamine and pacing stresses [30–34] have all been studied for this purpose (Table 9.1). The methodologies of these non-exercise approaches are described in Chapters 4 and 5, and each method has particular benefits and disadvantages. Atrial pacing has proven to be very safe (as the stress may be terminated instantly), but it remains invasive and uncomfortable, even with the recent development of combined transesophageal pacing and imaging. Dobutamine stress may provide unique data about myocardial viability (see Chapter 10), but its safety in a large

Table 9.1. Estimation of post-infarction prognosis by exercise echocardiography.

Author	Reference	n	Stress	Timing post-MI	WMA sens	ST sens
Jaarsma	27	43	Treadmill	3W	77%	55%
Applegate	28	67	Treadmill	2W	63%	38%
Ryan	29	40	Treadmill	2–3W	80%	55%
Iliceto	30	83	Atrial pacing	<3W	65%	32%
Bolognese	31	104	Dipyridamole	1–2W	45%	32%
Bosco	32	78	Dipyridamole	1–2W	76%	29%

AP = angina pectoris, MI = myocardial infarction, sens = sensitivity, spec = specificity, WMA

population of patients early after infarction remains to be established. Dipyridamole may produce transient but uncomfortable side-effects, but appears to be safe and is probably the main alternative to exercise echocardiography. All three have proven effective for the detection of multivessel disease and have provided acceptable positive and negative predictive values for the subsequent development of cardiac events. A large multicenter study using dipyridamole (the EPIC study) is in progress [35]; preliminary results suggest that the combined ability of echocardiography to document both resting dysfunction and ischemia may be translated into the ability to stratify risk accordingly (Figure 9.2).

The superiority of stress echocardiography over the stress ECG for the assessment of prognosis in post-infarction patients has been further supported in a series of 401 patients [36]. Of these subjects, those with both exercise ECG and dipyridamole echocardiography being positive for ischemia accounted for the only cardiac deaths, together with a 51% event rate over a 3 year follow-up. Patients with positivity at neither test had a 7% event rate. Of the remainder, there was a 21% event rate in the group with a positive stress ECG only, and a 40% event rate in those with a positive stress echocardiogram only. Moreover, the ability of stress echocardiography to distinguish heterozonal from homozonal ischemia causes stress echocardiography to be significantly more sensitive and specific than the stress ECG for the definition of multivessel disease [37].

While both stress perfusion scintigraphy and stress echocardiography are more effective than the stress ECG for post-infarct prognostication, few data are available to compare them. As discussed in Chapter 7, flow heterogeneity may be evident with milder, prognostically less important disease than that which causes regional ischemic dysfunction. Preliminary data suggest that these different mechanisms may account for some differences in the prognostic power of each test. McNeill [38] compared dipyridamole stress echocardiography and MIBI-SPECT in patients after recent myocardial infarction. Dipyridamole echocardiography proved the most accurate for the prediction of subsequent hard events, largely because of a higher positive predictive value.

In summary, the results of stress echocardiography for prognostication after infarction are encouraging. The acceptance of stress echocardiography

WMA sens	ST sens	Events	Mean follow-up
95%	67%	MI, AP	12 weeks
80%	76%	Death, MI, CABG	11 months
95%	65%	Death, MI, AP, CABG	6–10 months
92%	78%	MI, AP	14 months
74%	70%	Death, MI, AP, CABG	13 months
92%	92%	Death, MI, AP	

= wall motion abnormality.

as a means of post-infarct risk stratification has thus far been tempered by the small size of studies, with few "hard" end-points, and the extensive data validating the use of scintigraphic techniques for risk stratification. However, the data becoming available from the EPIC study promises to circumvent these reservations [35]. Nonetheless, the advent of thrombolytic therapy has significantly diminished the event-rate in post-infarct patients, and the relative cost-effectiveness of all these techniques will have to be re-addressed in the thrombolytic era.

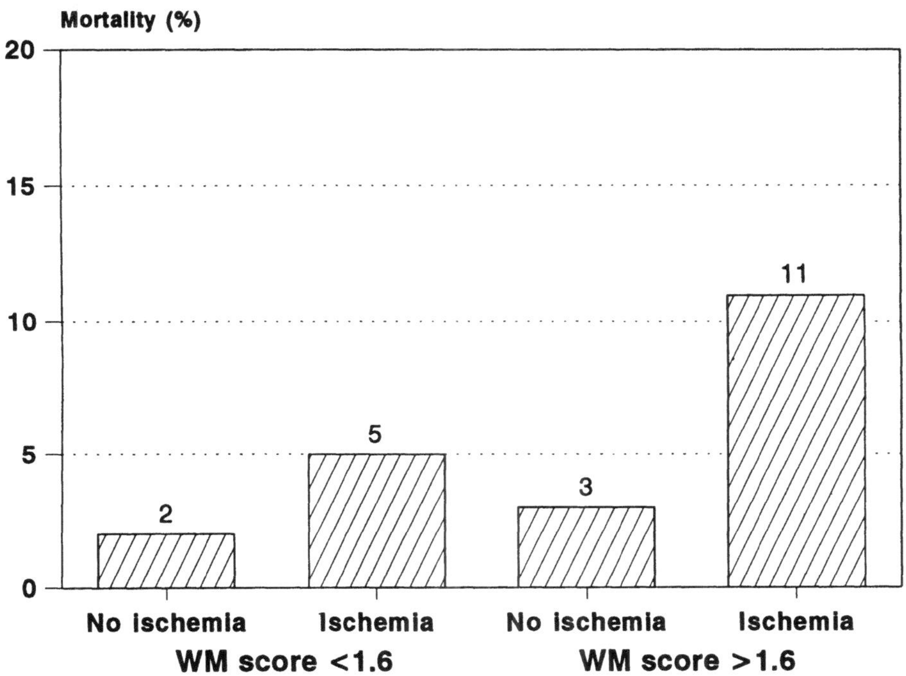

Figure 9.2. Prediction of post-infarction mortality (over 15 ± 10 months), based upon normal or abnormal resting LV function (wall motion score index less or greater than 1.6), and the absence or presence of ischemia.

Table 9.2. Prediction of perioperative cardiac events with stress echocardiography in patients

Author	Ref	n	Stress	Sensitivity	Specificity	PV+
Tischler	60	109	Dipyridamole	7/8 (88%)	99/101 (98%)	7/9 (78%)
Marwick	61	67	Dipyridamole	12/15 (80%)	46/52 (88%)	12/18 (67%)
Lane	62	57	Dobutamine	4/4 (100%)	19/34 (56%)	4/19 (21%)
Lalka	63	60	Dobutamine	10/12 (83%)	28/48 (58%)	10/30 (33%)
Davila-Roman	64	91	Db + atropine	17/17 (100%)	68/74 (92%)	17/23 (74%)
Poldermans	65	131	Db + atropine	15/15 (100%)	96/116 (83%)	15/35 (43%)

AP = angina pectoris, Db = dobutamine, CABG = coronary bypass surgery, LVF = left value of a positive test, PV − = predictive value of a negative test.

9.3 Prediction of Cardiac Events in Patients Undergoing Major Non-cardiac Surgery

9.3.1 *Background*

Coronary atherosclerosis is frequently present in patients with atherosclerotic disease elsewhere [39], and the occurrence of peri-operative coronary events has therefore been studied extensively in combination with major vascular surgery. Cardiac events are the leading cause of perioperative death [40–42], and severe coronary disease is also the major contributor to late deaths after vascular surgery. Due to the inactivity conferred by these diseases, myocardial ischemia may not be provoked by increased myocardial oxygen demand in the daily life of such patients. Thus, about 15% of those undergoing vascular surgery have occult coronary artery disease [39], which may first present with peri-operative myocardial infarction, serious arrhythmias or death. For these reasons, attempts have been made to identify patients with coronary disease and to revascularize selected patients to reduce the risk of vascular surgery [43]. Available tools for risk stratification include clinical evaluation, exercise stress testing, pharmacologic stress testing (usually in combination with echocardiographic or scintigraphic imaging), and coronary angiography. The latter is too expensive for screening all vascular patients, and will not be discussed further.

Clinical risk stratification in this situation is of value as a preliminary measure. Classical surgical risk scores [44] reflect the prognosis of general surgical populations (where coronary disease is less prevalent), and have been shown to have limited efficacy in predicting "at risk" patients among those with a high prevalence of cardiac disease [45]. A more specific clinical evaluation of coronary risk may be of some value [46]. In contrast to other situations of clinical uncertainty about the diagnosis of coronary disease, exercise stress testing is not routinely useful to precipitate ischemia, because limitation of exercise capacity due to cerebrovascular events or limb ischemia may compromise the sensitivity of the exercise ECG [47], even in combination with perfusion scintigraphy, nuclear ventriculography or echocardio-

undergoing vascular surgery.

PV−	Accuracy	Events
99/100 (99%)	106/109 (97%)	MI, AP
46/49 (94%)	58/67 (87%)	MI, AP, CABG
19/19 (100%)	23/38 (61%)	Death, MI, CABG
28/30 (93%)	38/60 (63%)	Death, MI, AP, CABG
68/68 (100%)	85/91 (93%)	MI, AP, CABG
96/96 (100%)	111/131 (85%)	MI, AP, LVF

ventricular failure, MI = myocardial infarction, PV + = predictive

graphy [48–51]. Use of a non-exercise stress is therefore appropriate in this population.

Dipyridamole stress myocardial perfusion scintigraphy is currently the most widely accepted pharmacologic stress testing methodology for risk stratification in these patients. This test is highly sensitive for the detection of coronary stenoses – so that a negative dipyridamole thallium test reliably implies the absence of disease and has a high negative predictive value for the absence of cardiac events after surgery [52–54]. The positive predictive value of scintigraphy for the prediction of cardiac events has been less satisfactory. In the above studies, the frequency of events in those with positive scans ranges from 33 to 44% [46,53,54], with the highest frequency (50%) in the study of Boucher [52]. In part, these results reflect the suboptimal specificity of thallium perfusion imaging, particularly in unselected (often elderly) populations, which include patients at high risk of false positive perfusion scintigrams such as those with left bundle branch block and left ventricular hypertrophy [55,56]. Paradoxically, the high sensitivity of dipyridamole thallium imaging may also contribute to these results, as patients with moderate coronary disease are readily identified, even though they are less likely than those with severe disease to suffer a cardiac event.

9.3.2 *Stress Echocardiographic Methods for Risk Stratification in Vascular Surgery Patients*

As stress echocardiography is potentially widely available and relatively inexpensive, it would be attractive as a technique for risk stratification in vascular surgery patients. Indeed, preliminary data suggest that pharmacological stress echocardiography is effective in this setting (Table 9.2).

As discussed in Chapter 5, dipyridamole induces ischemia by creating coronary steal. This usually requires the presence of severe or extensive stenoses [57], and hence the technique is relatively insensitive to mild or single-vessel disease [58], and is thereby less sensitive for the diagnosis of coronary disease than is perfusion scintigraphy [59]. Dipyridamole echocardiography has been used for risk stratification prior to vascular surgery

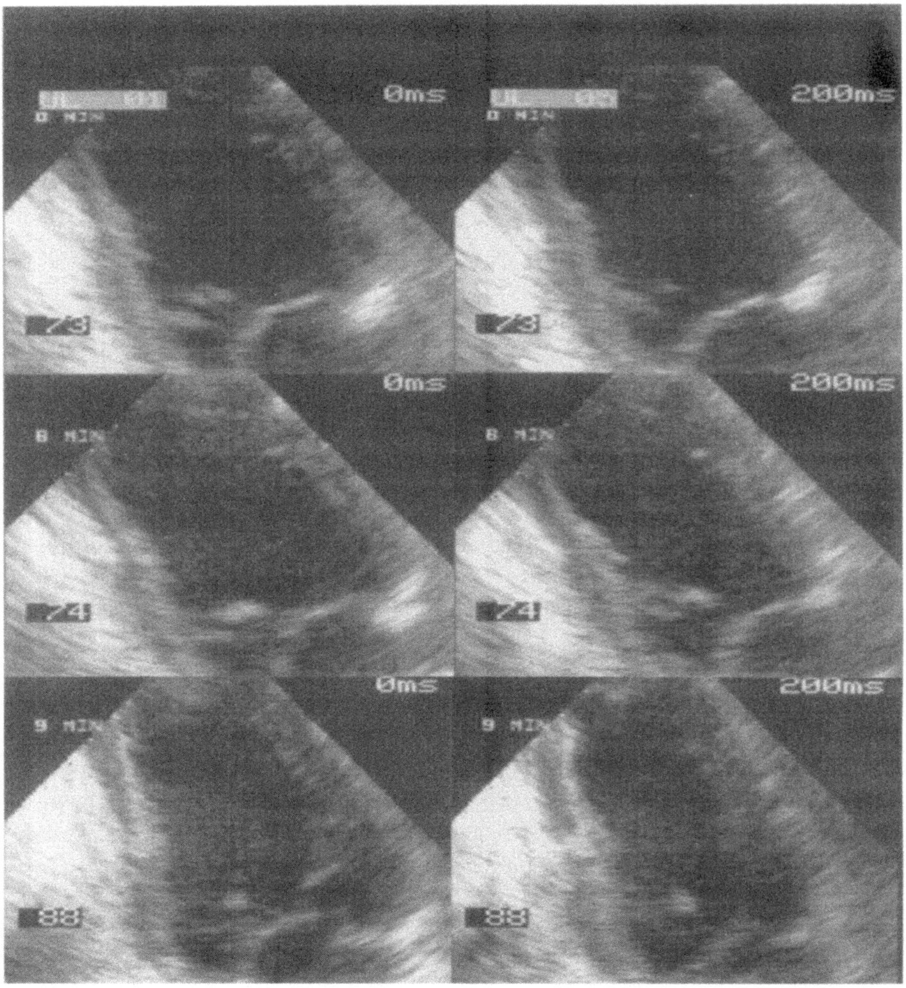

Figure 9.3. Diastolic (left) and systolic 4–chamber views at rest, after low and high-dose dipyridamole echocardiography in a patient undergoing vascular surgery. The lateral wall (arrows) contracts normally at rest (top), and becomes hypokinetic (middle) and then dyskinetic (bottom) indicating ischemia. At angiography, the patient was found to have circumflex and right coronary disease, and underwent myocardial revascularization prior to vascular surgery.

(Figure 9.3). The high positive predictive value (78%) of this test reported by Tischler [60] in a group of 109 vascular surgery patients may reflect the relatively selective detection of multivessel disease, and therefore, of patients who are more likely to develop complications from the stress and hemo-

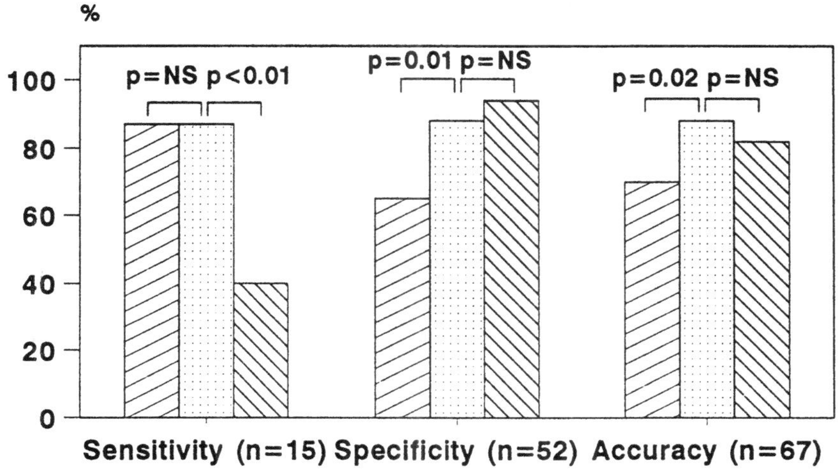

	Sensitivity (n=15)	Specificity (n=52)	Accuracy (n=67)
DpTl	87	65	70
DpEcho	87	88	88
DpECG	40	94	82

DpTl DpEcho DpECG

n=67 pts

Figure 9.4. Correlation of peri-operative events (see text) with ischemia identified by electrocardiography, echocardiography and thallium-SPECT during dipyridamole stress.

dynamic challenges of vascular surgery. Moreover, the lower sensitivity of dipyridamole echocardiography for milder coronary disease did not compromise its negative predictive value (99%).

The specificity of vasodilator stress echocardiography in an unselected clinical population [59] appears to exceed that of tomographic perfusion scintigraphy (SPECT). In view of both higher specificity and the selective detection of multivessel (prognostically more important) disease, dipyridamole echocardiography might be expected on theoretical grounds to offer a better positive predictive value for risk stratification than thallium imaging. Only one study [61] has compared the prognostic ability of both tests in the same patients undergoing vascular surgery (Figure 9.4). Among 67 patients undergoing dipyridamole stress echocardiography and thallium-SPECT, vascular surgery, and follow-up, 15 had a cardiac endpoint (perioperative ischemia or myocardial infarction, or cancellation of surgery for cardiac concerns and/or pre-operative coronary revascularization). Patients with endpoints could not be predicted reliably on clinical grounds, but correlated with the detection of ischemia by echocardiography or thallium-SPECT. The sensitivity of thallium-SPECT for the prediction of events was not significantly different from that of echocardiography (67% vs 80%), but the latter was more sensitive than angina and ST segment changes alone (sensitivity 40%, p = 0 01) The predictive value of a positive thallium test was 36% – less than with echocardiography (67%, p = NS) or ST segment changes and/or angina (66%, p = NS) The specificity of thallium SPECT (65%) was less than that of echocardiography (88%, p 0 01%) or angina and ST segment depression (94%, p = 0 01) The predictive value of a negative result was high with all tests 87%, 94%, and 84% with thallium SPECT, echocardiography and ST segment changes, respectively The accuracy of thallium-SPECT (66%) was less than that of echocardiography (87%, p = 0 02) and ST changes and angina (82%, P = 0 05) The results of this study suggest that dipyridamole echocardiography is a feasible, and more specific alternative to thallium SPECT for the prediction of cardiac events in patients undergoing vascular surgery

Dobutamine stress echocardiography has also been used for peri-operative risk stratification [62–65] In these series, the predictive value of a negative dobutamine echocardiogram in patients undergoing vascular surgery has been high, reflecting the high sensitivity of dobutamine echocardiography Indeed, on multivariate testing, the presence of ischemia provoked by dobutamine echocardiography increased the risk of an event by 42-fold [65] Even in those patients with a positive test who have surgery cancelled, there is a high prevalence of events at follow-up However, while this method is more sensitive than the vasodilator stress approach for the prediction of coronary disease, the principal difference in sensitivity is patients with single vessel disease [59] Such individuals may have good collateral flow and a good contractile reserve, making them less likely to suffer a major cardiac event at the time of surgery Not surprisingly, the positive predictive value of dobutamine echocardiography for peri-operative cardiac events has been somewhat lower, consistent with the identification of milder coronary disease, and correlating with the experience of dipyridamole thallium imaging

In summary, the various pharmacologic stress-imaging combinations share a high negative predictive value for the identification of patients unlikely to suffer peri-operative complications Further data are required but preliminary results suggest that dipyridamole echocardiography may be the test of choice for risk stratification in patients undergoing vascular surgery, because of the high predictive value of a positive test

9.4 Conclusion

The three situations discussed in this chapter – the group undergoing diagnostic stress, the post infarction population, and the high-risk operative patients – all provide evidence of the prognostic power of stress echocardiography In general, the predictive power of a negative test is very high, reflecting the high sensitivity of stress echocardiography for coronary disease of greater than moderate severity. The predictive power of a positive test, while much lower (because not all "at risk" patients suffer events) appears to be greater in some situations than that of perfusion scintigraphy. Such comparisons between non-invasive imaging approaches, in respect of their ability to predict disease endpoints, will attract increasing attention in the current cost-cutting environment in health care.

References

1. Marcus M, Skorton S, Johnson, Collins, Harrison, Kerber R. Visual estimates of percent diameter coronary stenosis: "A battered gold standard". J Am Coll Cardiol 1988;11:882–5.
2. Klocke F. Measurements of coronary blood flow and degree of stenosis: Current clinical implications and continuing uncertainties. J Am Coll Cardiol 1983;1:31–41.
3. Kannel WB, Feinlieb M. Natural history of angina pectoris in the Framingham study: Progress and survival. Am J Cardiol 1972;29:154–61.
4. Taylor HA, Deumite NJ, Chaitman BR *et al.* Asymptomatic left main coronary artery disease in the coronary artery surgery study (CASS) registry. Circulation 1989;79:1171–9.
5. Proudfit WL, Kramer JR, Goormastic M, Loop FD. Survival of patients with mild angina or myocardial infarction without angina; A comparison of medical and surgical treatment. Br Heart J 1988;59:641–7.
6. Armstrong WF, O'Donnell J, Ryan T, Feigenbaum H. Effect of prior myocardial infarction and extent and location of coronary disease on accuracy of exercise echocardiography. J Am Coll Cardiol 1987;10:531–8.
7. Andrade MJ, Landi P, Michelassi C, Malasoma M, Gimelli A, and EPIC investigators. Dipyridamole echocardiography in left main coronary stenosis [abstract]. Echocardiography 1993 (in press).
8. Weiner DA, Ryan TJ, McCabe CH *et al.* Prognostic importance of a clinical profile and exercise test in medically treated patients with coronary artery disease. J Am Coll Cardiol 1984;3:772–80.
9. Brown KA. Prognostic value of thallium-201 myocardial perfusion imaging: A diagnostic tool comes of age. Circulation 1991;83:363–81.
10. Lee KL, Pryor DB, Pieper KS *et al.* Prognostic value of radionuclide angiography in medically treated patients with coronary artery disease. A comparison with clinical and catheterization variables. Circulation 1990;82:1705–17.
11. Corday S, Martin S, Areeda J, Hajduczki I. Prognostic value of treadmill echocardiography in patients with chest pain and positive stress ECG [abstract]. Circulation 1988;78:II–272.
12. Diamond GA. Reverend Bayes' silent majority: An alternative factor affecting sensitivity and specificity of exercise electrocardiography. Am J Cardiol 1986;57:1175–80.
13. Pamelia FX, Gibson RS, Watson DD *et al.* Prognosis with chest pain and normal thallium-201 exercise scintigrams. Am J Cardiol 1985;55:920–6.
14. Sawada SG, Ryan T, Conley MJ, Corya BC, Feigenbaum H, Armstrong WF. Prognostic value of a normal exercise echocardiogram. Am Heart J 1990;120:49–54.
15. Picano E, Severi S, Michelassi C *et al.* Prognostic importance of dipyridamole-echocardiography test in coronary artery disease. Circulation 1989;80:450–7.
16. Marcovitz PA, Bach DS, Shayna VL, Armstrong WF. An abnormal dobutamine echocardiogram predicts death and myocardial infarction in the year following study [abstract]. Circulation 1992;86:I–789.

17. Luria MH, Debanne SM, Osman MI. Long-term follow-up after recovery from acute myocardial infarction. Arch Intern Med 1985;145:1592–5.
18. Multicenter Postinfarction Research Group. Risk stratification and survival after myocardial infarction. N Engl J Med 1983;309:331–6.
19. Nishimura RA, Reeder GS, Miller FA *et al.* Prognostic value of predischarge 2-dimensional echocardiogram after acute myocardial infarction. Am J Cardiol 1984;53:429–32.
20. Silverman KJ, Becker LC, Bulkley BH *et al.* Value of early thallium-201 scintigraphy for predicting mortality in patients with acute myocardial infarction. Circulation 1980;61:996–1003.
21. Theroux P, Waters DD, Halphen C, Debaisieux JC, Mizgala HF. Prognostic value of exercise testing soon after myocardial infarction. N Engl J Med 1989;30:341–52.
22. Gibson RS, Watson DD, Craddock GB *et al.* Prediction of cardiac events after uncomplicated myocardial infarction: A prospective study comparing predischarge exercise thallium-201 scintigraphy and coronary angiography. Circulation 1983;68:321–36.
23. Nicod P, Corbett JR, Firth BG *et al.* Prognostic value of resting and submaximal exercise radionuclide ventriculography after acute myocardial infarction in high risk patients with single and multivessel disease. Am J Cardiol 1985;52:30–6.
24. DeBusk RF. Specialized testing in recent acute myocardial infarction. Ann Intern Med 1989;110:470–81.
25. Norris RM, Caughey DE, Deeming LW, Mercer CJ, Scott PJ. Coronary prognostic index for predicting survival after recovery from acute myocardial infarction. Lancet 1970;ii:485–91.
26. Candell-Riera J, Permanyer-Miralda G, Castell J *et al.* Uncomplicated first myocardial infarction: Strategy for comprehensive prognostic studies. J Am Coll Cardiol 1991;18:1207–19.
27. Jaarsma W, Visser CA, Funke Kupper AJ, Res JC, Van Eenige MJ, Roos JP. Usefulness of two-dimensional exercise echocardiography shortly after myoardial infarction. Am J Cardiol 1986;57:86–90.
28. Applegate RJ, Dell'Italia LJ, Crawford MH. Usefulness of two-dimensional echocardiography during low-level exercise testing early after uncomplicated acute myocardial infarction. Am J Cardiol 1987;60:10–4.
29. Ryan T, Armstrong WF, O'Donnell JA, Feigenbaum H. Risk stratification after acute myocardial infarction by means of exercise two-dimensional echocardiography. Am Heart J 1987;114:1305–16.
30. Iliceto S, Caiati C, Ricci A *et al.* Prediction of cardiac events after uncomplicated myocardial infarction by cross-sectional echocardiography during transesophageal pacing. Int J Cardiol 1990;28:95–104.
31. Bolognese L, Sarasso G, Aralda D, Bongo SA, Rossi L, Rossi P. High dose echocardiography test early after uncomplicated acute myocardial infarction: Correlation with exercise testing and coronary angiography. J Am Coll Cardiol 1989;14:357–63.
32. Bosco M, Gandolfo N, Belli R, Parigi A, Schon W. Prognostic value of echocardiography with high-dose dipyridamole after recent uncomplicated myocardial infarction. G Ital Cardiol 1991;21:15–22.
33. Berthe C, Pierard LA, Hiernaux M *et al.* Predicting the extent and location of coronary artery disease in acute myocardial infarction by echocardiography during dobutamine infusion. Am J Cardiol 1986;58:1167–72.
34. Mannering D, Cripps T, Leech G *et al.* The dobutamine stress test as an alternative to exercise testing after acute myocardial infarction. Br Heart J 1988;59:521–6.
35. Landi P, Orlandini A, Chiarella F *et al.* The prognostic value of rest and stress echocardiography early after uncomplicated acute myocardial infarction: The first 995 patients of the EPIC study [abstract]. J Am Coll Cardiol 1993;21:441A.
36. Severi S, Michelassi C. Prognostic impact of stress testing in coronary artery disease. Circulation 1991;83(Suppl III):82–8.

37. Bolognese L, Sarasso G, Bongo AS *et al.* Stress testing in the period after infarction. Circulation 1991;83(Suppl III):32–7.
38. McNeill A, Slagboom T, Salustri A *et al.* Residual ischaemia after recent myocardial infarction: Comparison of high dose dipyridamole stress echocardiography and Tc-99 m MIBI SPECT [abstract]. Eur Heart J 1991;12:230.
39. Hertzer NR, Beven EG, Young JR *et al.* Coronary artery disease in peripheral vascular patients. A classification of 1000 coronary angiograms and results of surgical management. Ann Surg 1984;199:223–33.
40. Jamieson WR, Janusz MT, Miyagishima RT, Gerein AN. Influence of ischemic heart disease on early and late mortality after surgery for peripheral occlusive vascular disease. Circulation 1982;66:92–7.
41. Ennix CL, Lawrie GM, Morris GC *et al.* Improved results of carotid endarterectomy in patients with symptomatic coronary disease: An analysis of 1546 consecutive carotid operations. Stroke 1979;10:122–5.
42. Crawford ES, Bomberger RA, Glaeser DH *et al.* Aortoiliac occlusive disease: Factors influencing survival and function following reconstructive operation over a twenty-five year period. Surgery 1981;90:1055–66.
43. Foster ED, Davis KB, Carpenter JA *et al.* Risk of noncardiac operation in patients with defined coronary disease: The Coronary Artery Surgery Study (CASS) registry experience. Ann Thor Surg 1986;41:42–7.
44. Goldman L, Caldera DL, Nussbaum SR *et al.* Multifactorial index of cardiac risk in noncardiac surgical procedures. N Engl J Med 1977;297:845–50.
45. Takase B, Younis LT, Labovitz AJ *et al.* Comparison of the prognostic value of rest 2-dimensional echocardiography, dipyridamole stress thallium myocardial imaging, and clinical indices for perioperative cardaic events in major nonvascular surgical patients [abstract]. J Am Coll Cardiol 1992;19:101A.
46. Eagle KA, Singer DE, Brewster DC, Darling RC, Mulley AG, Boucher CA. Dipyridamole thallium scanning in patients undergoing vascular surgery. Optimizing preoperative evaluation of cardiac risk. JAMA 1987;257:2185–9.
47. Cumming GR. Yield of ischemic exercise electrocardiograms in relation to exercise intensity in a normal population. Br Heart J 1972;34:919–23.
48. Brady TJ, Thrall JH, Lo K *et al.* The importance of adequate exercise in the detection of coronary heart disease by radionuclide ventriculography. J Nucl Med 1980;21:1125–30.
49. Iskandrian AS, Heo J, Kong B, Lyons E. Effect of exercise level on the ability of thallium-201 tomographic imaging in detecting coronary artery disease: Analysis of 461 patients. J Am Coll Cardiol 1989;14:1477–86.
50. Marwick T, Nemec J, Pashkow F, Stewart WJ, Salcedo E. Accuracy and limitations of exercise echocardiography in a routine clinical setting. J Am Coll Cardiol 1992;19:74–81.
51. Leppo J, Boucher CA, Okada RD, Newell JB, Strauss HW, Pohost GM. Serial thallium-201 myocardial imaging after dipyridamole infusion: diagnostic utility in detecting coronary stenoses and relationship to regional wall motion. Circulation 1982;66:649–62.
52. Boucher CA, Brewster DC, Darling RC, Okada RD, Strauss HW, Pohost GM. Determination of cardiac risk by dipyridamole thallium imaging before peripheral vascular surgery. N Engl J Med 1985;312:389–94.
53. Eagle KA, Coley CM, Newell JB *et al.* Combining clinical and thallium data optimizes preoperative assessment of cardiac risk before major vascular surgery. Ann Intern Med 1989;110:859–66.
54. Leppo J, Plaja J, Gionet M, Tumolo J, Paraskos JA, Cutler BS. Noninvasive evaluation of cardiac risk before elective vascular surgery. J Am Coll Cardiol 1987;9:269–76.
55. DePuey EG, Guertler-Krawczynska E, Robbins WL. Thallium-201 SPECT in coronary disease patients with left bundle branch block. J Nucl Med 1988;29:1479–85.
56. DePuey EG, Guertler-Krawczynska E, Perkins JV, Robbins WL, Whelchel JD, Clements SD. Alterations in myocardial thallium-201 distribution in patients with chronic systemic

hypertension undergoing single-photon emission computed tomography. Am J Cardiol 1988;62:234–8.

57. Picano E. Dipyridamole echocardiography test: The historical background and the physiologic basis. Eur Heart J 1989;10:365–76.
58. Mazeika P, Nihoyannopoulos P, Joshi J, Oakley CM. Uses and limitations of high dose dipyridamole stress echocardiography for evaluation of coronary artery disease. Br Heart J 1992;67:144–9.
59. Marwick T, Willemart B, D'Hondt AM *et al.* Selection of the optimal non-exercise stress for the evaluation of ischemic regional myocardial dysfunction and malperfusion: Comparison of dobutamine and adenosine using echocardiography and Tc-99 m MIBI single photon emission computed tomography. Circulation 1993;87:345–54.
60. Tischler MD, Lee TH, Hirsch AT *et al.* Prediction of major cardiac events after peripheral vascular surgery using dipyridamole echocardiography. Am J Cardiol 1991;68:593–9.
61. Vincent M, Marwick T, D'Hondt AM *et al.* Prediction of perioperative events at vascular surgery: Selection of thallium scintigraphy or echocardiography with dipyridamole stress? [abstract]. Circulation 1992;86:I–790.
62. Lane RT, Sawada SG, Segar DS *et al.* Dobutamine stress echocardiography for assessment of cardiac risk before noncardiac surgery. Am J Cardiol 1991;68:976–7.
63. Lalka SG, Sawada SG, Dalsing MC *et al.* Dobutamine stress echocardiography as a predictor of cardiac events associated with aortic surgery. J Vasc Surg 1992;15:831–42.
64. Davila-Roman VG, Waggoner AD, Sicard GA, Geltman EM, Schechtman KB, Perez JE. Dobutamine stress echocardiography predicts surgical outcome in patients with an aortic aneurysm and peripheral vascular disease. J Am Coll Cardiol 1993;21:957–63.
65. Poldermans D, Fioretti PM, Forster T *et al.* Dobutamine stress echocardiography for assessment of perioperative cardiac risk in patients undergoing major vascular surgery. Circulation 1993;87:1506–12.

10. Echocardiographic Determination of Myocardial Viability

T. MARWICK and J-L. VANOVERSCHELDE

Regional myocardial dysfunction after myocardial infarction is not always due to irreversible damage to all involved tissue. Early after acute ischemic events, "stunning" (dysfunction despite normalization of coronary perfusion) resolves spontaneously [1]. Later after the event, dysfunction in viable tissue may be due to further episodes of stunning due to recurrent ischemia, or to chronic ischemia, which is often termed "hibernation" [2]. In the latter situations, resumption of normal function is contingent upon prevention of recurrent or ongoing ischemia, usually by myocardial revascularization.

The presence of viable myocardium may influence clinical decision-making with respect to the mode of revascularization, and possibly the decision to revascularize. The mode of revascularization may be altered if viable myocardium is identified in a region thought to be infarcted - in order to resupply such an additional territory, a multi-vessel angioplasty or bypass surgery may need to be considered in preference to a single-vessel angioplasty. Moreover, preliminary data are emerging to support the use of revascularization in patients with viable myocardium, who do not otherwise fulfill the usual symptomatic or prognostic indications for intervention. First, global ejection fraction [3] and the patient's overall functional capacity [4] may be enhanced by revascularization. Second, evidence is accumulating that such tissue is inherently unstable without revascularization, and is liable to further events [5,6]. The detection of viable myocardium is therefore clinically pertinent to both referral of patients for intervention, and the type of intervention.

10.1 Definition of "Viable Myocardium"

Some form of reference standard is required to define and compare the accuracies of techniques for predicting myocardial viability. Metabolic, contractile or global functional markers of myocardial viability have been utilized, without a concensus as to the most reliable methodology. Although used as a test to identify viable myocardium, metabolic markers of myocardial viability (see below) have been used as a reference standard in some studies. Such a design permits simultaneous performance of the test in question and the reference standard, precluding misleading results due to intercurrent events, or attrition of patients either because of failure to revascularize

T.H. Marwick, Stress Echocardiography, 163–178.

or failure to return for follow-up. However, this approach has the major disadvantage of being clinically impractical – patients are revascularized in order to improve the function of affected regions, rather than to reperfuse metabolically viable tissue – indeed, not all areas of perfusion-metabolism mismatch recover functionally. For these reasons, the use of metabolic imaging is unsatisfactory as a reference standard.

A more widely accepted definition of myocardial viability is the improvement of regional systolic function following myocardial revascularization. This approach requires patient follow-up after revascularization (usually at 3 months), in order to document whether regional function has improved, indicating viability. The use of a relevant clinical endpoint (regional function) outweighs the constraints imposed by performing a follow-up study.

In addition to the improvement in regional wall motion and thickening, improvement in global left ventricular function should also be considered in the definition of myocardial viability. Prognostic studies have indeed indicated that indices of global systolic function (such as end-systolic volume and ejection fraction) are strong predictors of survival in patients with chronic left ventricular dysfunction due to coronary artery disease [7]. In such patients, coronary revascularization by either bypass surgery or balloon angioplasty, may thus not only improve ventricular function, but also prolong survival. In addition, it has been shown that the degree of improvement in global left ventricular function following coronary revascularization was intimately related to the amount of salvageable myocardium [3]. This implies that some threshold amount of viable tissue is needed to impact on global left ventricular function and on prognosis. Thus, although the improvement of regional left ventricular function identifies the presence of viable myocardium, clinical decision-making may be dependent upon quantification of the amount available to produce an improvement in left ventricular function.

10.2 Approaches to the Detection of Myocardial Viability

The conventional techniques used for the detection of myocardial viability include the absence of ECG Q-waves, the absence of regional left ventricular dysfunction, and "fixed" scintigraphic perfusion defects. Electrocardiographic Q-waves are not specific for infarction; they may be caused by ischemia, in which circumstance they may be reversible [8]. Such tissue may be erroneously identified as non-viable, a discrepancy which is particularly common following thrombolysis. Their presence correlates poorly with myocardial viability, assessed on metabolic grounds [9]. Regional left ventricular dysfunction may reflect myocardial stunning or hibernation rather than infarction, so that 30–40% of regions with pre-operative dysfunction will demonstrate enhancement of function after revascularization [10]. Thallium perfusion defects after stress, which fail to reverse on 4-hour redistribution images, do not preclude functional recovery after revascularization – either

PTCA [11] or surgery [12]. In summary, these conventional approaches for the definition of myocardial viability lack sufficient accuracy to be wholly satisfactory for routine clinical use.

Two new scintigraphic approaches have been applied to the problem of identifying viable infarct-zone tissue which is likely to recover function with revascularization. These include position emission tomography (PET) and thallium scintigraphy with thallium reinjection. Several approaches have been proposed to identify jeopardized but viable myocardium by use of PET. Because depressed regional contractile performance secondary to ischemia reflects underlying derangement of myocardial perfusion and metabolism, flow and metabolic imaging has been the focus of much attention. The hallmark of viable myocardium using the FDG technique is demonstration of a "metabolism perfusion mismatch" of persisting glucose uptake in malperfused regions [13]. Results of studies in patients with left ventricular dysfunction due to chronic coronary artery disease have indicated that positron imaging with F-18 deoxyglucose or with C-11 acetate accurately predicts the presence of viable myocardium within dysfunctional areas. Using the FDG approach, myocardial viability can be detected with sensitivities in the range of 75–85% and specificities of 78–92% [3,14,15]. However, the FDG techniques greatly overestimate both the amount and the extent of viable myocardium in patients with previous myocardial infarction [16,17]. Although the suboptimal positive predictive accuracy of PET in these studies may reflect inadequate revascularization, graft closure or restenosis, it may also be a manifestation of the exquisite sensitivity of FDG imaging for small (usually subepicardial) portions of myocardium which may not contribute materially to contraction when revascularized. Therefore, because many patients with coronary artery disease and poor left ventricular ejection fraction have sustained one or more previous myocardial infarctions in the past, assessment of myocardial viability with PET and FDG alone may offer insufficient diagnostic accuracy for appropriate clinical management and decision making.

The alternative method for the assessment of myocardial viability using PET is based upon the evaluation of regional myocardial oxygen consumption and absolute blood flow. Because of the aerobic nature of cardiac contraction, assessment of myocardial oxidative metabolism with PET and C-11 acetate has been recently proposed to evaluate the potential for functional recovery after revascularization. Under experimental conditions of ischemia followed by reperfusion, maintenance of oxidative metabolism has been shown to be an important determinant of viability and to portend the recovery of contractile function following reperfusion [18]. In patients with chronic coronary artery disease with [17] or without [19] previous myocardial infarction, it was recently shown that maintenance of oxidative metabolism was a prerequisite to functional recovery after coronary revascularization. Evaluation of absolute levels of regional perfusion to dysfunctional myocardium may also be helpful in distinguishing viable from nonviable myocardium without recourse to metabolic imaging. Preliminary data suggest that segments that will eventually recover function upon coronary revascularization have higher absolute levels of myocardial blood flow [20] and a greater transmural proportion of the myocardium that is "perfusable" [21] compared with segments that remain dysfunctional postoperatively.

Myocardial viability may also be assessed by measurement of membrane retention of cationic tracers. As concentration of these agents within the myocyte is against an electrochemical gradient, cell viability is a prerequisite for their concentration within the cell. While reduced tracer delivery in comparison with normal regions may cause "perfusion defects" on immediate post-exercise images, viable myocardium continues to concentrate the tracer over subsequent hours, as the agent continues to perfuse the tissue. Eventually, the "perfusion defect" appears to resolve as increasing amounts of tracer are concentrated in the region of interest [22]. In patients with severe coronary stenosis [23], this process is constrained by reduced tracer delivery, explaining why failure to "redistribute" at 4 hours does not necessarily connote non-viable tissue. The problems posed by delayed redistribution may be circumvented by allowing for a longer redistribution time such as 24 hours (but this is often impractical clinically), or reinjecting thallium in order to augment the delivery of the tracer [24,25]. The latter method correlates well with viability estimated by position emission tomography [26]. Limited data [25] suggest that thallium reversibility after thallium reinjection predicts enhancement of regional function after revascularization, with 87% sensitivity and 100% specificity.

Preliminary data with both dobutamine and dipyridamole suggest that the responses of regional left ventricular function to either of these agents may be effective in the detection of viable myocardium. Although all stress methodologies may be used to identify peri-infarct ischemia and heterozonal ischemia, no data exist in relation to the detection of viable myocardium with exercise stress.

10.3 Diagnosis of Viable Myocardium Using Dobutamine Echocardiography

Experimental models of myocardial stunning generally involve occlusion of a coronary artery, followed after a variable time by resumption of normal coronary flow. Even after an ischemic period of only 20 minutes, regional function may remain impaired for up to 6 hours. Provided that the myocardium is viable and non-ischemic [27–31], the severity of this dysfunction may be temporarily ameliorated by sympathomimetic agents – isoproterenol, dopamine and dobutamine. The mechanism of this response is unclear, but appears to be truly inotropic and unrelated to alterations in loading conditions.

In contrast with myocardial stunning, there is no valid experimental model for chronic hibernation. In contrast to experimental models which purely involve myocardial stunning, the clinical pathophysiology of chronic regional dysfunction due to coronary disease is more complex, involving both post-ischemic dysfunction and ongoing reduction of coronary flow. It was initially proposed that hibernation resulted from chronic or ongoing myocardial ischemia. Recent observations suggest that it could instead arise from repetitive episodes of myocardial stunning, eventually resulting in prolonged post-ischemic dysfunction [32]. Whatever the mechanisms, myocardial hibernation in humans is associated with marked ultrastructural alterations of the myocytes, which includes a profound loss of myofilaments and contractile material [32]. It should therefore not be surprising if the hibernating tissue was not as responsive to inotropic stimulation as purely stunned myocardium. The hibernating segments may also show no or a very limited residual coronary flow reserve, which should also limit their ability to increase function upon inotropic stimulation. The clinical implications of these findings are that stunned myocardium, which is probably predominant in the early post-infarction setting, might be detected using dobutamine echocardiography, while hibernating myocardium, which may be preponderant later after infarction, might be less responsive to this test.

Conventional dobutamine protocols (see Chapter 4) have been combined with echocardiography for the determination of myocardial viability. However, the interpretation of functional responses for the purpose of determination of myocardial viability generally involves responses to low doses of dobutamine (Figure 10.1). Combinations of augmentation of function at low dose, with deterioration of function at high dose, may be used to identify non-viable tissue, viable myocardium supplied by a stenosed or non-stenosed artery, or simply myocardial ischemia (Table 10.1).

The applicability of dobutamine testing to patients studied early (<2 weeks) after myocardial infarction has been confirmed clinically. Using nuclear ventriculography, Sadler [33], showed that the detection of viable myocardium (defined by responsiveness to isopreterenol) correlated with the presence of patent infarct-related arteries in post-thrombolysis patients. The ejection fraction in such patients rose by $14 \pm 1\%$, in contrast to $6 \pm 1\%$ in those with occluded vessels. Correlation of dobutamine responsiveness with follow-up findings was obtained by Barilla [34]. In this study of a selected group of patients found to have dobutamine responsive regions after "incomplete" infarction (comprising patients with non Q-wave infarcts, and patients with infarction treated with thrombolytic therapy), regions predicted to be viable by dobutamine responsiveness were found to improve after subsequent revascularization. Non-revascularized segments responded to dobutamine, but showed less improvement at follow-up (Figure 10.2), suggesting that these regions were still ischemic, and implying that viable, but dysfunctional and ischemic (hibernating) regions could still be dobutamine responsive. These data have been reproduced in a less selected group of post-thrombolysis patients by Smart [35], who showed that improvement of the wall motion score index with low-dose dobutamine had a 71% sensitivity for its

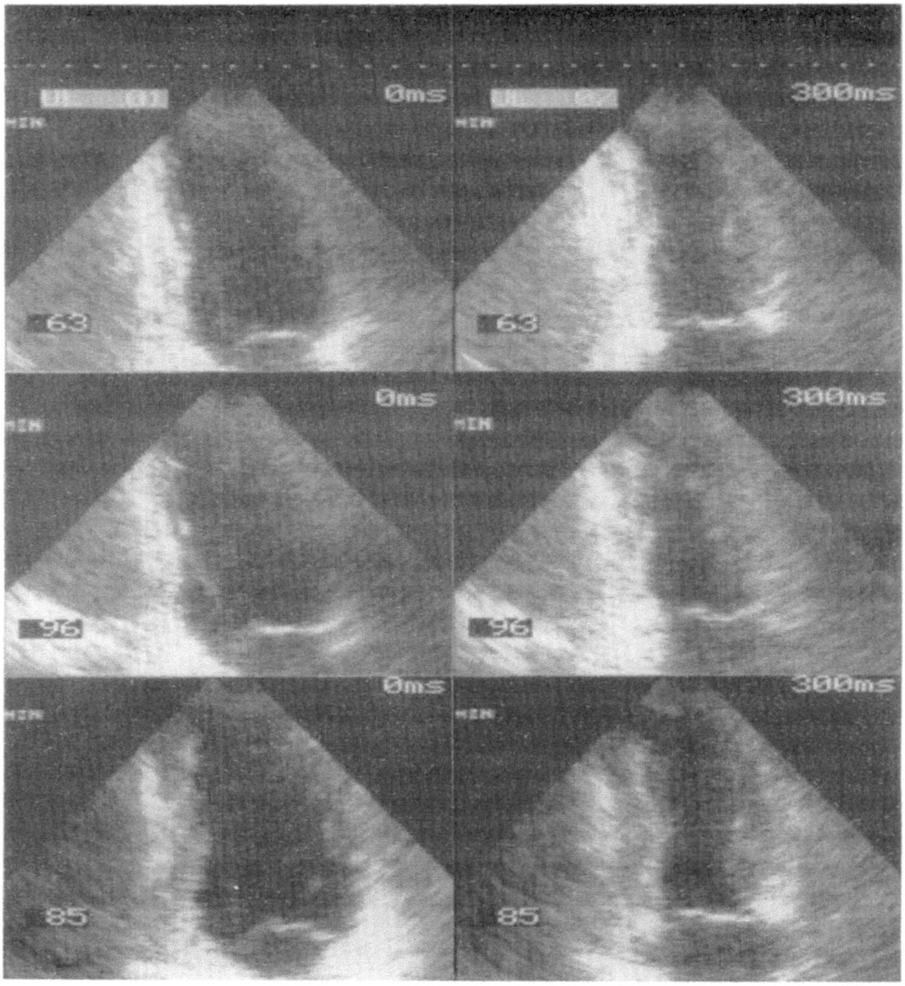

Figure 10.1. Diastolic (left) and systolic 2–chamber images and traced drawings at rest (top), 5 mcg/kg/minute and 10 mcg/kg/minute (bottom) of dobutamine. The patient has anterior akinesis

recovery at follow-up, while the absence of an improvement had a specificity of 74% for failure to improve at follow-up. These investigators also found that improvement at high-doses of dobutamine (20 mcg/kg/min) was not a reliable predictor of recovery.

The issue of stunning and hibernation in relation to dobutamine responsiveness has also been examined by Pierard [36]. In this study, the prediction of myocardial viability using low-dose dobutamine echocardiography was compared with its prediction using positron emission tomography in 17 patients after thrombolysis. Early after admission, the diagnosis of viability

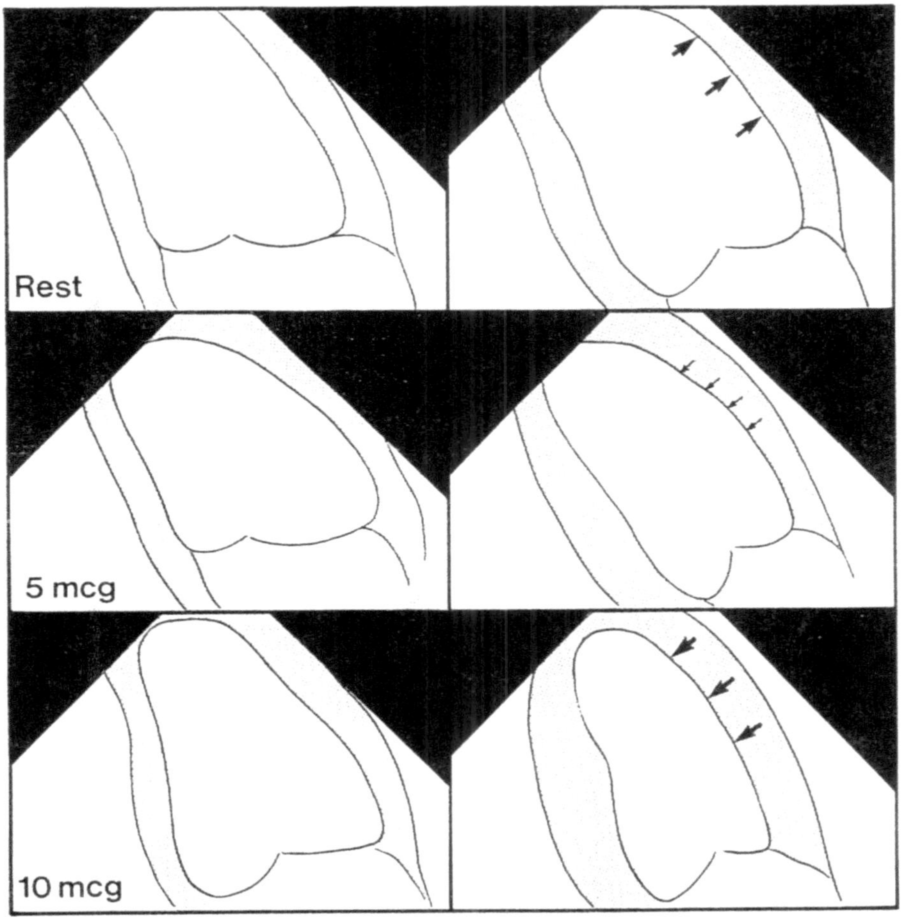

(arrows) at rest, with progressive thickening of the basal- and mid-anterior segments in response to dobutamine, denoting myocardial viability.

Table 10.1. Interpretation of dobutamine echocardiography for the diagnosis of myocardial viability in patients with abnormal resting function.

Diagnosis	Rest	Low dose Db	Peak dose Db
Ischemia – mild	Normal/abnormal	No change	Reduced
Ischemia – severe	Normal/abnormal	Reduced	Reduced
Viable – patent IRA	Abnormal	Improved	Improved
Viable – occluded IRA	Abnormal	Improved (?)	Reduced
Infarction	Abnormal	No change	No change

Db = dobutamine, IRA = infarct-related artery.

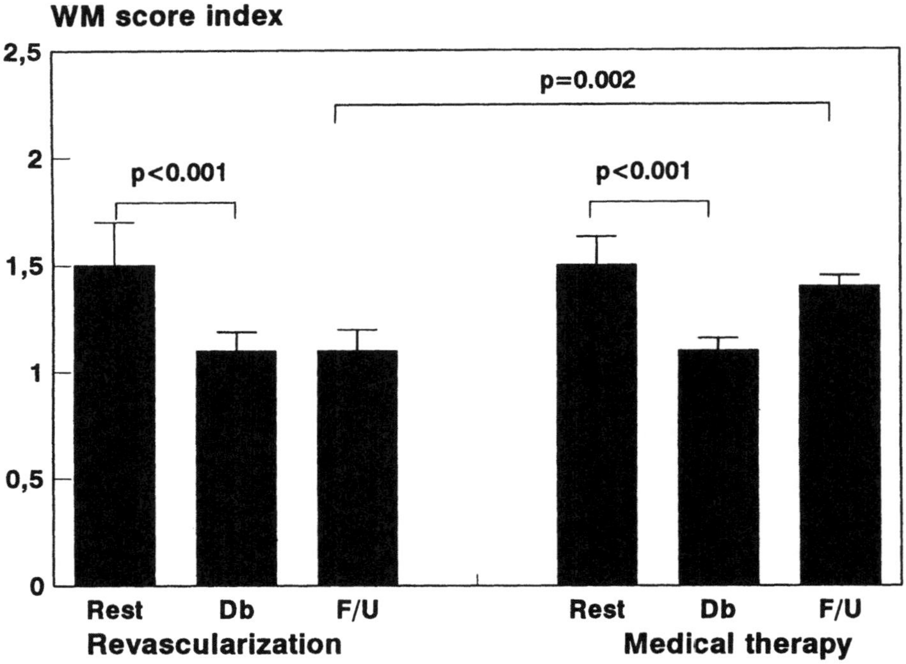

Figure 10.2. Comparison of echocardiographic wall motion score index in revascularized and non-revascularized patients at baseline (rest), after low-dose dobutamine (Db), and follow-up (F/U) in patients with viable myocardium after "incomplete" myocardial infarction (see text). Modified from Barilla [34].

correlated in 79% of segments. However, of the patients responding to dobutamine, only those with preservation of regional perfusion (who did not require revascularization) showed functional recovery at follow-up (Figure 10.3). In contrast, patients having regions predicted to be viable on the basis of persistent metabolic activity despite reduced flow did not demonstrate functional recovery at follow-up, even though all but one demonstrated dobutamine responsiveness. These data support the hypothesis that both stunned and hibernating myocardium are responsive to dobutamine. However, the response of hibernating myocardium appears to be less predictive of recovery than the equivalent response in stunned tissue. This conclusion must be tempered by the small numbers involved, with 2 of the six patients with hibernation not being revascularized.

While existing data suggest that augmentation of regional function in response to dobutamine stress may predict myocardial viability in the early post-infarct period, few data are available to support or refute the efficacy of dobutamine testing for the prediction of myocardial viability later after myocardial infarction. Preliminary data have addressed the accuracy of regional dobutamine responsiveness for the prediction of functional recovery of abnormal function due to revascularization late after infarction [37]. In 36

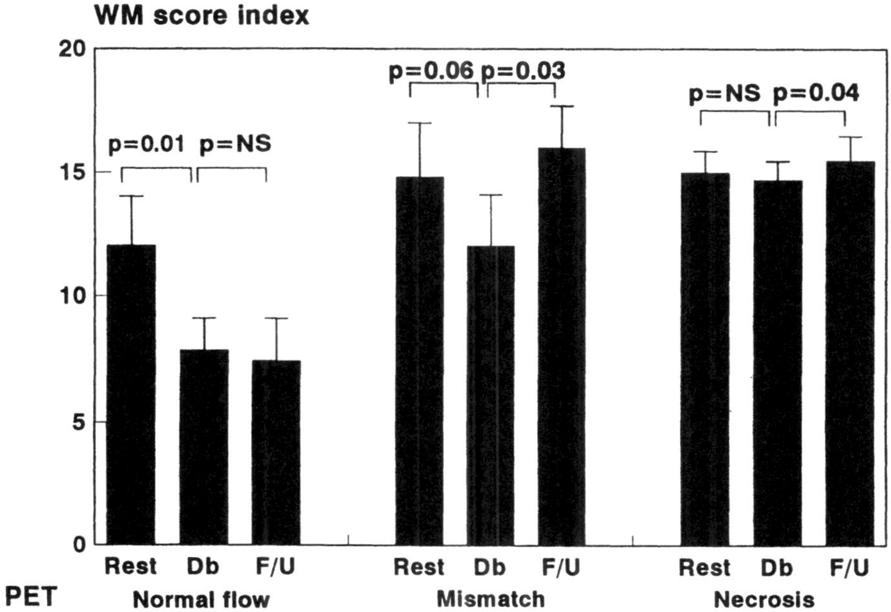

Figure 10.3. Alteration of wall motion score index (a lower index implying better function) in response to dobutamine (Db) and follow-up (F/U) in patients with normal perfusion, perfusion-metabolism mismatch, and necrotic myocardium by PET criteria. Modified from Pierard [36].

patients who underwent revascularization by angioplasty (n = 17) or bypass surgery (n = 19), we evaluated recovery of regional function 5 ± 3 months after revascularization. A total of 201 segments showed akinesis or dyskinesis before revascularization. Sixty of these segments (29%) improved function after revascularization and were accordingly considered as viable, while the remaining 141 segments showed no or minimal improvement after revascularization and were therefore considered as nonviable. Of the 60 viable segments, 48 had improved function during infusion of low-dose dobutamine before revascularization (sensitivity 80%). Of the 141 nonviable segments, 111 had shown no or trivial functional improvement with dobutamine (specificity 79%). The overall accuracy of dobutamine echocardiography, on a segmental basis, was 80%. The predictive value of a positive test was 62% and that of a negative test 89%. We also considered the accuracy of the test to predict improvement in both regional and global left ventricular function in an individual patient analysis. Twenty-one patients had viable myocardium in 2 segments or more, and did not deteriorate global function after revascularization (group 1). The remaining 15 patients had none or minimally viable tissue, and had further increased in both end-diastolic and end-systolic volume after revascularization (group 2). Both groups were similar with respect to pre-revascularization ejection fraction and exercise capacity. Dobutamine echocardiography correctly identified 20 of 21 patients from group 1 (95%),

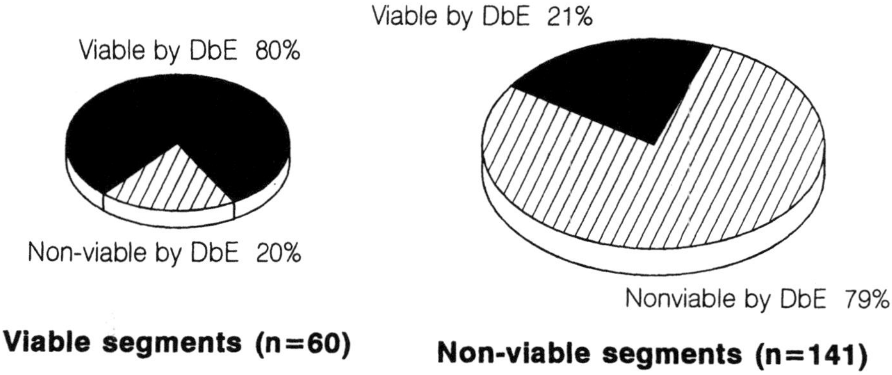

Figure 10.4. Accuracy of dobutamine echocardiography for prediction of myocardial viability, defined by improvement of regional function after revascularization [37].

while it failed to improve function in 11 of 15 patients of group 2 (73%). Overall, 31 of 36 patients (86%) were correctly categorized by dobutamine echocardiography. These data suggest that dobutamine responsiveness is a highly sensitive test for the prediction of viability with good specificity and negative predictive value.

10.4 Dobutamine Echocardiography vs Reinjection Thallium Imaging for Identification of Viability

The feasibility and apparent accuracy of dobutamine echocardiography for the definition of myocardial viability has led some authors to question whether it may be able to compete with scintigraphic approaches for the diagnosis of viable myocardium. In our initial approach to this comparison, we compared the concordance between low-dose dobutamine echocardiography and reinjection Tl-201 imaging in 21 patients, at an interval of 22 ± 37 months after infarction [38]. Regions of interest were specified by the presence of regional dysfunction and/or a resting perfusion defect subtended by the infarct-related artery; viability (at Tl imaging) was defined by filling in of a resting defect at either the 4 hour or the Tl reinjection images, and viability (at echocardiography) was defined by residual contractile function, or functional improvement or deterioration (ischemia) in response to dobutamine. Of 185 segments, both were in agreement regarding the diagnosis of viable myocardium in 90 and its absence in 35, giving a concordance of 68%, with approximately equal numbers of the remainder identified as viable by each technique. Using the Tl results as the reference standard for diagnosis of viability, 43 segments were viable, for which echocardiography had a sensitivity of 70%, and 64 were non-viable, in which echocardiography showed a specificity of 55%.

In a follow-up study, Marzullo and coworkers [39] studied 14 patients 35 ± 24 weeks after the acute event, and analyzed the relation between radioisotopic (rest Tl-201 or rest Tc-99 m sestamibi scans) and echocardiographic markers of viability as well as the relative sensitivity and specificity of these methods in predicting the recovery of function after revascularization. Of the 75 dysfunctional myocardial segments identified at baseline on resting echocardiograms, 49 (65%) showed improved wall motion at the follow-up study, 11 ± 2 weeks after revascularization, and were considered as viable. At pre-revascularization dobutamine echocardiography, 82% of these viable segments improved function by at least one full grade during dobutamine echocardiography, while 92% of the nonviable segments failed to improve wall motion. These results favorably compared with the sensitivity (86%) and specificity (92%) of delayed thallium imaging in the same patients.

We have also analyzed the concordance between low-dose (5 to 10 mcg/kg/min) dobutamine echocardiography and thallium-201 exercise-redistribution-reinjection scintigraphy in 33 patients with regional left ventricular dysfunction, most [31–33] with previous myocardial infarction [40]. The patients were studied at an average of 5 ± 2 months after the index event. Their mean ejection fraction was 40 ± 14%. All patients underwent resting pre and post-revascularization two-dimensional echocardiography. Myocardial viability was defined as an improvement in regional wall motion score by at least one full grade in 2 adjacent segments. Twenty-one patients improved regional wall motion after revascularization, while the remaining 12 patients did not. Pre-revascularization criteria for viability were: by thallium-201 reinjection scintigraphy, a preserved or only moderate decrease of thallium uptake (>50% of maximal activity), by dobutamine echocardiography, an improvement in regional wall motion score by at least one full grade in two adjacent segments. The positive predictive value of thallium reinjection for viable myocardium was 86%, similar to that of low-dose dobutamine echocardiography (87%). The negative predictive values for the two tests were also similar, respectively 87% and 90%. These preliminary data suggest that, late after myocardial infarction, dobutamine echocardiography appears to have similar accuracy to thallium reinjection scintigraphy for the diagnosis of viable myocardium.

10.5 Diagnosis of Viable Myocardium Using Dipyridamole Echocardiography

Sympathomimetic agents are not alone in their ability to induce transient improvements in the function of stunned myocardium. Both dipyridamole and papaverine [41] have been shown to enhance both segmental shortening and load-independent indices of ventricular function in stunned myocardium, and the same may be true of adenosine (Figure 10.5). The mechanisms responsible for these effects remain ill-defined. An indirect sympathomimetic

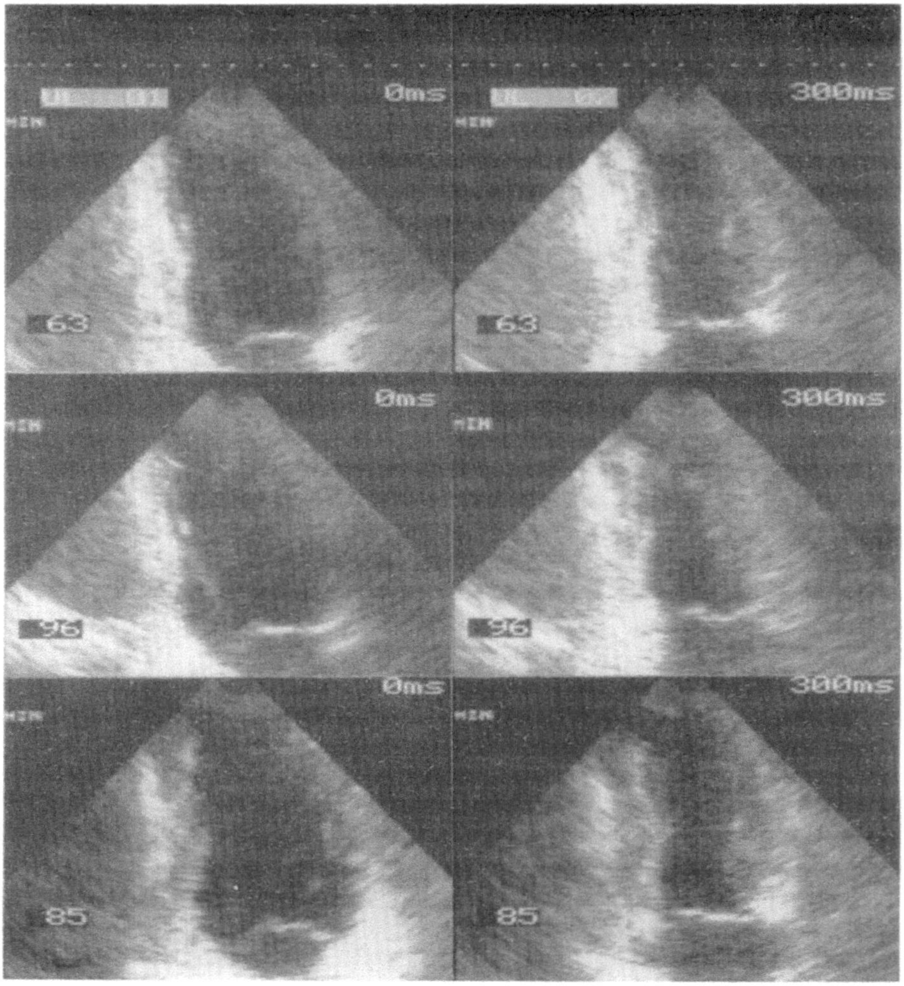

Figure 10.5. Diastolic (left) and systolic 2-chamber views and equivalent traced images at rest (top) and during low- and high-dose (bottom) adenosine echocardiography. Resting antero-apical akinesis resolves at low dose (myocardial arrows), indicating viability, with recurrence at high dose (endocardial arrows), suggesting ischemia.

effect, occurring as a response to dipyridamole-induced ischemia is possible. Augmentation of myocardial blood volume may increase contractility by mechanisms analogous to the Frank-Starling relationship. Finally, if tissue is not stunned but chronically ischemic, coronary perfusion may be enhanced by these vasodilators.

Clinically, dipyridamole stress echocardiography has been shown to effec-

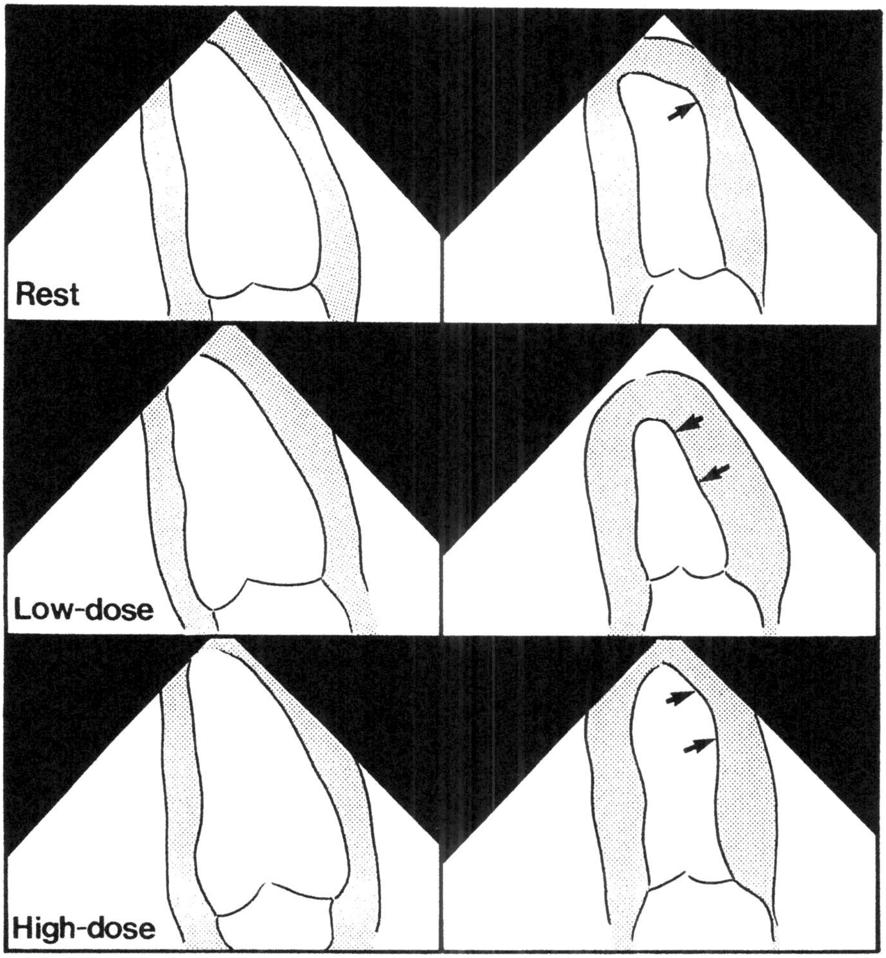

tively identify both heterozonal and peri-infarct ischemia in patients after myocardial infarction [42]. Recent data presented by Picano [43] suggest that this test may also be able to identify viable myocardium. In 22 patients, 15 of whom had an old (>3 months) infarction, dipyridamole echocardiography (using a standard high-dose protocol) and rest/late redistribution thallium imaging were performed, with follow-up echocardiography being obtained in 15 patients. Echocardiographic evidence of myocardial viability was defined by an augmentation of regional function during the hyperkinetic phase of the dipyridamole response; at thallium imaging, it was defined by regional activity >55%. Using the thallium criteria as a reference standard for the interpretation of 80 aynergic segments, dipyridamole echocardiography had a sensitivity of 81%, and a specificity of 96%. Using recovery of function after revascularization as the reference standard, dipyridamole echocardiography had a sensitivity of 79% in 19 segments showing an improvement in function, and 87% in 39 segments which failed to improve function.

10.6 Conclusion

Enhancement of regional left ventricular function is not the main outcome sought by intervention, which is really aimed at improving global left ventricular function and the overall functional state of the patient. These endpoints may be measured by ventricular volumes and ejection fraction, or exercise capacity after revascularization – all of which require analysis on a patient rather than a regional basis. There is a paucity of functional follow-up data in general, and none available with either dobutamine echocardiography or thallium reinjection techniques. In summary, while enhancement of regional function is an accepted endpoint for myocardial viability, there may be a disparity (currently undefined) between the ability of different tests of viability to predict recovery in global functional indices.

The place of stress echocardiography in the assessment of patients following myocardial infarction currently centers upon the detection of residual myocardial ischemia (see Chapter 9) – either in another coronary territory (manifest as "heterozonal asynergy") or in the same territory (peri-infarct ischemia). Preliminary data suggest that the revascularization of viable myocardium after myocardial infarction may be beneficial for prognosis. Thus, the most appropriate test for patients after myocardial infarction may be one which is able to detect heterozonal ischemia, peri-infarct ischemia and viable myocardium. However, the relative importance in the detection of viable tissue within the infarct site, in addition to residual ischemia, remains unresolved.

References

1. Kloner RA, Przyklenk K, Patel B. Altered myocardial states: The stunned and hibernating myocardium. Am J Med 1986;86(suppl 1A):14.
2. Rahimtoola SH. The hibernating myocardium. Am Heart J 1989;117:2113.
3. Tillisch J, Brunken R, Marshall R *et al.* Reversibility of cardiac wall-motion abnormalities predicted by positron tomography. N Engl J Med 1986;314:884.
4. Marwick T, Nemec JJ, Lafont A, Salcedo EE. Improvement of exercise capacity after revascularization: Prediction by post-exercise F-18 deoxyglucose positron emission tomography. Am J Cardiol 1992;69:854.
5. Eitzman D, Al Aouar Z, Kanter HL *et al.* Clinical outcome of patients with advanced coronary disease after viability studies with positron emission tomography. J Am Coll Cardiol 1992;20:559.
6. Lee K, Marwick T, Cook S *et al.* Failure to revascularize patients with hibernating myocardium is strongly associated with adverse cardiac events. Circulation 1992;86:I–107.
7. White HD, Norris RM, Brown MA, Brandt PWT, Whitlock RML, Wild CJ: Left ventricular

end-systolic volume as the major determinant of survival after recovery from myocardial infarction. Circulation 1987, 76:44–51

8. Zeft HJ, Friedberg HD, King JF, Manley JC, Huston JH, Johnson WD. Reappearance of anterior QRS forces after coronary bypass surgery; an electrovectorcardiographic study. Am J Cardiol 1975;36:163.
9. Brunken R, Tillisch J, Schwaiger M *et al.* Regional perfusion, glucose metabolism, and wall motion in patients with chronic electrocardiographic Q wave infarctions: evidence for persistence of viable tissue in some infarct regions by positron emission tomography. Circulation 1986;73:951.
10. Brundage BH, Massie BM, Botvinick EH. Improved regional ventricular function after successful surgical revascularization. J Am Coll Cardiol 1984;3:902.
11. Liu P, Keiss MC, Okada RD *et al.* The persistent defect on exercise Thallium imaging and its fate after myocardial revascularization: does it represent scar or ischemia? Am Heart J 1985;110:996.
12. Gibson RS, Watson DD, Taylor GJ *et al.* Prospective assessment of regional myocardial perfusion before and after coronary revascularization surgery by quantitative thallium-201 scintigraphy. J Am Coll Cardiol 1983;1:804.
13. Schelbert HR, Buxton D. Insights into coronary artery disease gained from metabolic imaging. Circulation 1988;78:496.
14. Tamaki N, Yonekura Y, Yamashita K *et al.* Positron emission tomography using fluorine-18 deoxyglucose in evaluation of coronary artery bypass grafting. Am J Cardiol 1989;64:860.
15. Marwick T, MacIntyre WJ, Lafont A, Nemec J, Salcedo E. Metabolic response of hibernating and infarcted myocardium to revascularization: A follow-up study of perfusion, function and metabolism. Circulation 1992;85:1347.
16. Schwaiger M, Brunken R, Grover-McKay M *et al.* Regional myocardial metabolism in patients with acute myocardial infarction assessed by positron emission tomography. J Am Coll Cardiol 1986;8:800–8.
17. Gropler RJ, Siegel BA, Sampathkumaran K *et al.* Dependence of recovery of contractile function on maintenance of oxidative metabolism after myocardial infarction. J Am Coll Cardiol 1992;19:989–97.
18. Weinheimer CJ, Brown MA, Nohara R, Perez JE, Bergmann SR. Functional recovery after reperfusion is predicted on recovery of myocardial oxidative metabolism. Am Heart J 1993;125:939–49.
19. Gropler RL, Geltman EM, Sampathkumaran K *et al.* Functional recovery after coronary revascularization for chronic coronary artery disease is dependent on maintenance of oxidative metabolism. J Am Coll Cardiol 1992;20:569–77.
20. Grandin C, Essamri B, Vanoverschelde J-L *et al.* Flow and metabolics correlates of functional recovery after anterior ischemia or infarction [abstract]. Circulation 1991;84:II–89.
21. De Silva R, Yamamoto Y, Rhodes CG *et al.* Preoperative prediction of the outcome of coronary revascularization using positron emission tomography. Circulation 1992;86:1738–42.
22. Beller GA, Pohost GM. Mechanisms for Tl-201 redistribution after transient myocardial ischemia. Circulation 1977;56:141.
23. Gutman J, Berman DS, Freeman M *et al.* Time to completed redistribution of thallium-201 in exercise myocardial scintigraphy: Relationship to the degree of coronary artery stenosis. Am Heart J 1983;106:989.
24. Kiat H, Berman DS, Maddahi J *et al.* Late reversibility of tomographic myocardial Tl-201 defects: An accurate marker of myocardial viability. J Am Coll Cardiol 1988;12:1456.
25. Dilsizian V, Rocco TP, Freedman NM, Leon MB, Bonow RO. Enhanced detection of ischemic but viable myocardium by the reinjection of thallium after stress-redistribution imaging. N Engl J Med 1990;323:141.
26. Bonow RO, Dilsizian V, Cuocolo A, Bacharach SL. Identification of viable myocardium in patients with chronic coronary artery disease and left ventricular dysfunction: Comparison

of thallium scintigraphy with reinjection and PET imaging with F-18 deoxyglucose. Circulation 1991;83:26.

27. Mercier JC, Lando U, Kanmatsuse K *et al.* Divergent effects of inotropic stimulation on the ischemic and severely depressed reperfused myocardium. Circulation 1982;66:397–403.
28. Buda AJ, Zotz RJ, Gallagher KP. The effect of inotropic stimulation on normal and ischemic myocardium after coronary occlusion. Circulation 1987;76:163–72.
29. Ellis SG, Wynne J, Braunwald E, Henschke CI, Sandor T, Kloner RA. Response of reperfusion-salvaged, stunned myocardium to inotropic stimulation. Am Heart J 1984;107:13–9.
30. Bolli R, Zhu WX, Myers ML, Hartley CJ, Roberts R. Beta-adrenergic stimulation reverses post-ischemic myocardial dysfunction without producing subsequent functional deterioration. Am J Cardiol 1985;56:946.
31. Mohaved A, Reeves WC, Rose GC, Wheeler WS, Jolly SR. Dobutamine and improvement of regional and global left ventricular dysfunction in coronary artery disease. Am J Cardiol 1990;66:365–7.
32. Vanoverschelde JLJ, Wijns W, Depre C *et al.* Mechanisms of chronic regional postischemic dysfunction in humans: New insights from the study of non-infarcted collateral dependent myocardium. Circulation 1993;87:1513–23.
33. Satler LS, Kent KM, Fox LM *et al.* The assessment of contractile reserve after thrombolytic therapy for acute myocardial infarction. Am Heart J 1986;111:821–5.
34. Barilla F, Gheorghiade M, Alam M, Khaja F, Goldstein S. Low-dose dobutamine in patients with acute myocardial infarction identifies viable but not contractile myocardium and predicts the magnitude of improvement in wall motion abnormalities in response to coronary revascularization. Am Heart J 1991;122:1522–31.
35. Smart SC, Sawada SG, Ryan T *et al.* Dobutamine echocardiography predicts recovery after thrombolysis in myocardial infarction [abstract]. Circulation 1990;82:III–75.
36. Pierard LA, De Landsheere Berthe C, Rigo P, Kulbertus HE. Identification of viable myocardium by echocardiography during dobutamine infusion in patients with myocardial infarction after thrombolytic therapy: Comparison with positron emission tomography. J Am Coll Cardiol 1990;15:1021–31.
37. Vanoverschelde J-L, Marwick T, d'Hondt A-M, Baudhuin T, Wijns W, Melin JA: Delineation of myocardial viability with low-dose dobutamine stress-echocardiography in patients with chronic ischemic left ventricular dysfunction [abstract]. Circulation 1993;88:I–111.
38. Marwick T, Baudhuin T, Willemart B, D'Hondt AM, Wijns W, Melin J. Direct comparison of thallium reinjection scintigraphy and dobutamine stress echocardiography for the diagnosis of viable myocardium in patients late after myocardial infarction [abstract]. Eur Heart J 1992;13(Suppl):44.
39. Marzullo P, Parodi O, Reisenhofer B *et al.* Value of rest thallium-201/technetium-99 m sestamibi scans and dobutamine echocardiography for detecting myocardial viability. Am J Cardiol 1993;71:166–72.
40. Melin JA, Marwick T, Baudhuin T, De Kock M, d'Hondt A-M, Vanoverschelde J-L. Assessment of myocardial viability with thallium-201 imaging and dobutamine echocardiography: A comparative analysis [abstract]. Circulation 1993;88:I–535.
41. Stahl LD, Aversano TR, Becker LC. Selective enhancement of function of stunned myocardium by increased flow. Circulation 1986;74:843–51.
42. Bolognese L, Sarasso G, Aralda D, Bongo AS, Rossi l, Rossi P. High dose dipyridamole echocardiography early after uncomplicated acute myocardial infarction: Correlation with exercise testing and coronary angiography. J Am Coll Cardiol 1989;14:357–63.
43. Picano E, Marzullo P, Gigli G *et al.* Identification of viable myocardium by dipyridamole-induced improvement in regional left ventricular function assessed by echocardiography in myocardial infarction and comparison with thallium scintigraphy at rest. Am J Cardiol 1992;70:703–10.

Index

Developments in Cardiovascular Medicine

121. S. Sideman, R. Beyar and A.G. Kleber (eds.): *Cardiac Electrophysiology, Circulation, and Transport.* Proceedings of the 7th Henry Goldberg Workshop (Berne, Switzerland, 1990). 1991 ISBN 0-7923-1145-0
122. D.M. Bers: *Excitation-Contraction Coupling and Cardiac Contractile Force.* 1991 ISBN 0-7923-1186-8
123. A.-M. Salmasi and A.N. Nicolaides (eds.): *Occult Atherosclerotic Disease.* Diagnosis, Assessment and Management. 1991 ISBN 0-7923-1188-4
124. J.A.E. Spaan: *Coronary Blood Flow.* Mechanics, Distribution, and Control. 1991 ISBN 0-7923-1210-4
125. R.W. Stout (ed.): *Diabetes and Atherosclerosis.* 1991 ISBN 0-7923-1310-0
126. A.G. Herman (ed.): *Antithrombotics.* Pathophysiological Rationale for Pharmacological Interventions. 1991 ISBN 0-7923-1413-1
127. N.H.J. Pijls: *Maximal Myocardial Perfusion as a Measure of the Functional Significance of Coronary Arteriogram.* From a Pathoanatomic to a Pathophysiologic Interpretation of the Coronary Arteriogram. 1991 ISBN 0-7923-1430-1
128. J.H.C. Reiber and E.E. v.d. Wall (eds.): *Cardiovascular Nuclear Medicine and MRI.* Quantitation and Clinical Applications. 1992 ISBN 0-7923-1467-0
129. E. Andries, P. Brugada and R. Stroobrandt (eds.): *How to Face 'the Faces' of Cardiac Pacing.* 1992 ISBN 0-7923-1528-6
130. M. Nagano, S. Mochizuki and N.S. Dhalla (eds.): *Cardiovascular Disease in Diabetes.* 1992 ISBN 0-7923-1554-5
131. P.W. Serruys, B.H. Strauss and S.B. King III (eds.): *Restenosis after Intervention with New Mechanical Devices.* 1992 ISBN 0-7923-1555-3
132. P.J. Walter (ed.): *Quality of Life after Open Heart Surgery.* 1992 ISBN 0-7923-1580-4
133. E.E. van der Wall, H. Sochor, A. Righetti and M.G. Niemeyer (eds.): *What's new in Cardiac Imaging?* SPECT, PET and MRI. 1992 ISBN 0-7923-1615-0
134. P. Hanrath, R. Uebis and W. Krebs (eds.): *Cardiovascular Imaging by Ultrasound.* 1992 ISBN 0-7923-1755-6
135. F.H. Messerli (ed.): *Cardiovascular Disease in the Elderly.* 3rd ed. 1992 ISBN 0-7923-1859-5
136. J. Hess and G.R. Sutherland (eds.): *Congenital Heart Disease in Adolescents and Adults.* 1992 ISBN 0-7923-1862-5
137. J.H.C. Reiber and P.W. Serruys (eds.): *Advances in Quantitative Coronary Arteriography.* 1993 ISBN 0-7923-1863-3
138. A.-M. Salmasi and A.S. Iskandrian (eds.): *Cardiac Output and Regional Flow in Health and Disease.* 1993 ISBN 0-7923-1911-7
139. J.H. Kingma, N.M. van Hemel and K.I. Lie (eds.): *Atrial Fibrillation, a Treatable Disease?* 1992 ISBN 0-7923-2008-5
140. B. Ostadel and N.S. Dhalla (eds.): *Heart Function in Health and Disease.* Proceedings of the Cardiovascular Program (Prague, Czechoslovakia, 1991). 1992 ISBN 0-7923-2052-2
141. D. Noble and Y.E. Earm (eds.): *Ionic Channels and Effect of Taurine on the Heart.* Proceedings of an International Symposium (Seoul, Korea , 1992). 1993 ISBN 0-7923-2199-5
142. H.M. Piper and C.J. Preusse (eds.): *Ischemia-reperfusion in Cardiac Surgery.* 1993 ISBN 0-7923-2241-X
143. J. Roelandt, E.J. Gussenhoven and N. Bom (eds.): *Intravascular Ultrasound.* 1993 ISBN 0-7923-2301-7
144. M.E. Safar and M.F. O'Rourke (eds.): *The Arterial System in Hypertension.* 1993 ISBN 0-7923-2343-2
145. P.W. Serruys, D.P. Foley and P.J. de Feyter (eds.): *Quantitative Coronary Angiography in Clinical Practice.* With a Foreword by Spencer B. King III. 1994 ISBN 0-7923-2368-8

Developments in Cardiovascular Medicine

146. J. Candell-Riera and D. Ortega-Alcalde (eds.): *Nuclear Cardiology in Everyday Practice.* 1993 (in prep.) ISBN 0-7923-2374-2
147. P. Cummins (ed.): *Growth Factors and the Cardiovascular System.* 1993 ISBN 0-7923-2401-3
148. K. Przyklenk, R.A. Kloner and D.M. Yellon (eds.): *Ischemic Preconditioning: The Concept of Endogenous Cardioprotection.* 1993 ISBN 0-7923-2410-2
149. T.H. Marwick: *Stress Echocardiography.* Its Role in the Diagnosis and Evaluation of Coronary Artery Disease. 1994 ISBN 0-7923-2579-6
150. W.H. van Gilst and K.I. Lie (eds.): *Neurohumoral Regulation of Coronary Flow.* Role of the Endothelium. 1993 ISBN 0-7923-2588-5

Previous volumes are still available

KLUWER ACADEMIC PUBLISHERS – DORDRECHT / BOSTON / LONDON

MIX
Papier aus verantwortungsvollen Quellen
Paper from responsible sources
FSC® C105338

If you have any concerns about our products,
you can contact us on
ProductSafety@springernature.com

In case Publisher is established outside the EU,
the EU authorized representative is:
Springer Nature Customer Service Center GmbH
Europaplatz 3, 69115 Heidelberg, Germany

Printed by Libri Plureos GmbH
in Hamburg, Germany